HANDBOOK OF SCHOOL HEALTH

First edition	1885
Second edition	1886
Third edition	1892
Fourth edition	1899
Fifth edition	1904
Sixth edition	1910
Seventh edition	1915
Eighth edition	1923
Ninth edition	1928
Tenth edition	1940
Eleventh edition	1948
Twelfth edition	1954
Thirteenth edition	1962
Fourteenth edition	1969
Fifteenth edition	1975
Sixteenth edition	1984

HANDBOOK OF SCHOOL HEALTH

Issued by
THE MEDICAL OFFICERS OF SCHOOLS ASSOCIATION

SIXTEENTH EDITION
1984

 MTP PRESS LIMITED
a member of the KLUWER ACADEMIC PUBLISHERS GROUP
LANCASTER / BOSTON / THE HAGUE / DORDRECHT

Published in the UK and Europe by
MTP Press Limited
Falcon House
Lancaster, England

British Library Cataloguing in Publication Data

Medical Officers of Schools Association
    Handbook of school health. — 16th ed.
    1. School hygiene — Great Britain
    I. Title
    371.7'0941   LB3409.G/

    ISBN 0-85200-734-5

Published in the USA by
MTP Press
A division of Kluwer Boston Inc
190 Old Derby Street
Hingham, MA 02043, USA

Library of Congress Cataloging in Publication Data

Main entry under title:

Handbook of school health.

    Bibliography: p.
    Includes index.
    1. School hygiene – Great Britain – Handbooks, manuals, etc.   2. Communicable
diseases – Great Britain – Prevention.   I. Hoskins, Trevor, 1931 –   II. Medical
Officers of Schools Association. [DNLM: 1. Communicable disease control.   2.
School health services. WA 350 H236]
LB3409. G7H36 1984   371.7'1'0941   84-4420
ISBN 0-85200-734-5

Copyright © 1984 MTP Press Limited

Typeset by UPS Blackburn Limited, 76-80 Northgate, Blackburn, Lancashire.

Printed by Redwood Burn Limited, Trowbridge.

CONTENTS

PREFACE TO THE SIXTEENTH EDITION

Ever since the first slim edition of this Handbook was published 100 years ago, it has been a tradition for the preface to be contributed by the President of the day. I happen to combine that honour in MOSA's centenary year with the office of Honorary Editor, which gives me the responsibility for preparing this new edition for the press. By a coincidence, the same conjunction of offices occurred in 1975 when the President was Surgeon Captain Peter de Bec Turtle, an indefatigable worker for MOSA for the past quarter of a century, and one of three former editors who have been of immense value to me on the Handbook Committee. It was a great sadness that his already substantial contribution to this edition came to an abrupt end with his lamented death in August 1983.

If his edition in 1975 was the largest and most radically revised in the Handbook's history, it set the pace for equally radical changes in this the 16th edition. The Committee has decided to rearrange the chapters in a more logical order, and much of the material has been rewritten. In a departure from previous practice, I have undertaken the bulk of the rewriting myself, with cross-checking by the full committee. This should result, for better or for worse, in a greater consistency in style, with a correspondingly heavier personal responsibility for errors, omission and infelicities. An exception has been in Chapter 8, where we have taken the opportunity to have the section on outdoor activities rewritten by an expert in the field, Dr J. O. B. Rosedale, a member of the Council of MOSA. He was greatly helped in this by Mr Patrick Heffron, master in charge of outdoor activities at Marlborough College. When they came to consider the section on exposure and heat exhaustion they found it impossible to improve upon the pithy contribution to the last edition by the late

Colonel Charles McNeil, who at that time was medical officer to Sedbergh School following his retirement as medical officer to the Royal Military Academy, Sandhurst. I therefore make no apology for the abrupt change of style for two pages which stand as a fitting memorial to another contributor whose loss we have mourned since the last edition.

It is with great pleasure that I acknowledge help from a wide circle of colleagues and friends; some of these may not have been consciously aware that they were contributing to our Handbook. One of the important functions of our Association is its clinical meetings and lectures which are means of keeping our members up to date with modern practice and developments in centres of excellence. Inevitably this becomes reflected in MOSA policy and the advice to be found in these pages. Among many consultants who have influenced us in this way are Professor Tim Clark and Dr John Stark who modernized our approach to asthma at a memorable meeting in Cambridge in 1979, and Drs Marcia Wilkinson, Barbara Boucher and John Price who have talked to us, respectively, on the childhood and adolescent aspects of headache, diabetes and respiratory infection. Specific advice has been freely given by several colleagues from the Public Health Laboratory Service: Dr Joan Davies, Deputy Director; Dr Spence Galbraith and Dr Norman Noah, director and consultant epidemiologist, respectively, of the Communicable Disease Surveillance Centre; and Dr Christine Miller of the Epidemiological Research Laboratory. Increasing concern over sports injuries has been reflected in Chapter 7, and I am grateful to Mr John Carvell, consultant orthopaedic surgeon at Salisbury General Hospital, for reading the draft and advising on some changes, and to Mr R. S. G. Rixon, MCSP, for discussing with me the fruits of his long experience in treating sportsmen.

One of the advantages of working in a school like Christ's Hospital is the ease of access to advice from teachers in a variety of subjects. Mr Richard Youdale, Head of Classics, helped me to avoid some of the more offensive neologisms which have crept into medicine, Mr Glyn James, Head of Chemistry, kindly checked the technical details of the passage on disinfectants, and Mr Jim Endacott, Master in Charge of Rugby, demonstrated his continuing interest in injury prevention by his thorough review of the relevant passages. Through the good offices of Mr John Perry, Head of Craft and Design, the artwork for Figures 1–5 was kindly prepared by one of his O level pupils, Tim Brookes. The school dental surgeon, Mr Victor Wiffen, is a close colleague whose enthusiasm for prevention in dentistry is reflected in the text.

Despite all the advice of those with special knowledge, however, this Handbook is nothing if not the distillation of experience gained by the practising school doctors who make up our membership. In this respect it is the work of an industrious Handbook Committee whose members have given detailed thought to its content and presentation, and painstakingly revised and corrected the various drafts. I am deeply indebted to them, but the ultimate responsibility for the final version must, of course, rest with me. An increasing amount of knowledge of the epidemiology of illness and injury in schools has been gathered individually and corporately by MOSA, and much of this is incorporated in the book.

We have tried to steer the perilous course between too much and too little detail in our endeavour to keep this Handbook as a concise work of easy reference. At the same time, we have attempted to cover most of the questions that can arise in the work of the school doctor and his colleagues. In the words of the late Peter Turtle in the Preface to the 15th edition,

> 'We hope that the book will find its way into the hands not only of school doctors, but also school nurses, teachers, psychologists, social workers, administrators, and indeed all who are concerned in the health and welfare of young people. We stress the importance of good communications between the school doctor, his professional colleagues in both teaching and medical professions inside and outside the school and perhaps, above all, the parents, whose children are his professional responsibility.'

Previous editions carried an editorial note to the effect that 'the alternative title headmistress may be understood when the title headmaster has been used', with similar treatment of assistant teachers and pupils. We have tried to incorporate a less sexist approach in this edition, but the English language is not easily bent to this purpose, and we must again explain that on occasions the personal pronoun of either sex must be taken to include both sexes, rather than litter the text with 'he-or-she's and 'his-or-her's. Although men outnumber women on our editorial committee we hope we can be exonerated of bias.

I gratefully acknowledge the advice of Dr John Wall of the Medical Defence Union. The extracts from *Health Education in Schools, The developmental progress of infants and young children* and the School Premises Regulations 1981 are reproduced with the permission of the Controller of Her Majesty's Stationery Office, the height and weight charts with the permission of the editor of *Archives of Disease in Childhood,* and material from Tanner's *Growth at Adolescence* with the permission of Blackwell Scientific Publications Ltd. Tables 1 and 2 are adapted from Welsby's *Infectious Diseases* with the permission of the publishers, MTP Press Ltd. The extract from Anna Freud's article on Adolescence is reproduced with the permission of International Universities Press, Inc., publishers of *The Psychoanalytic Study of the Child*. The tables in Appendix G first appeared in the *British Journal of Sport and Medicine,* and are reprinted with the editor's permission. I also acknowledge a generous donation from SKF Laboratories towards secretarial expenses.

Finally, I should like to express my thanks to our new publishers for their co-operation and patience, and my heartfelt appreciation of the work of Mrs June Rixon who has shouldered single-handed the burden of deciphering my manuscript, typing, retyping and preparing the final copy for the press.

TREVOR HOSKINS
President of MOSA 1983–1984
Honorary Editor

11 Chandos Street
Cavendish Square
London W1
January 1984

PREFACE TO THE FIRST EDITION

In bringing this Code of Rules before the general public and the Medical and Scholastic professions in particular, the Medical Officers of Schools Association desire to say a few words as to its compilation.

On the formation of the Association in 1884 one of the most urgent matters which forced itself to the front, as claiming immediate attention, was the need for the general adoption of more definite rules for guarding our great educational establishments from the outbreak and spread of preventible infectious disease.

With this object an attempt was made to ascertain the rules and customs which are at present enforced in such cases, by circulating to every school of any importance in the country an elaborate series of questions covering the ground of this inquiry.

The replies thus obtained proved very interesting, and contained much valuable material; at the same time they revealed wide differences of procedure in different institutions when dealing with the same conditions of disease, and, in some instances, a considerable laxity of precaution. Nothing could more clearly demonstrate the necessity for some definite and generally recognised standard of School Hygiene than the curiously divergent character of many of the answers furnished in response to our paper of questions on the commoner epidemic diseases.

In the course of their deliberations on the information thus collected, the Association have embodied opinions and suggestions from many special authorities on the several questions dealt with. It is hoped that the result of these labours may prove no less useful to parents and guardians, who deal with the home life of the children, than to the school authorities, since without the sympathy and intelligent co-operation of the former no real progress can be made in this great department of preventive medicine, which is fraught with so much benefit to the community at large.

The Medical Officers of Schools Association cannot allow this Code to go forth to the public without placing on record the great debt of gratitude which they owe to their indefatigable Secretary, Dr Aldersmith, the Medical Officer of Christ's Hospital. This Code is to a very large extent based on the valuable paper on *"The Preventive Treatment of Infectious Diseases in Public and High Schools,"* read by him at the Conference on School Hygiene, at the International Health Exhibition. The extensive correspondence involved in communicating with a very large number of schools and of individuals in all parts of the Kingdom has been entirely in his hands; upon him devolved the heavy labour of comparing and collating the replies received from the various authorities consulted; and upon him, too, has fallen the duty of preparing this work for the press.

G. J. H. EVATT, MD,
Surgeon-Major (later Surgeon-General), Army Medical Staff,
President, MOSA

Woolwich
January, 1885

THE HANDBOOK COMMITTEE

H. G. Barnes, MB BS, FRCGP. Medical Officer to the Royal Grammar School, Newcastle upon Tyne.

J. H. D. Briscoe, MA, MB BChir, D Obst RCOG, MRCGP. Medical Officer to Eton College and St George's School, Windsor Castle.

Joan D. K. Ferreira, MRCS LRCP, DHMSA. Sessional Clinical Medical Officer, Richmond, Twickenham and Roehampton District Health Authority; Medical Officer, Lady Eleanor Holles School, Hampton.

T. W. Hoskins, MA, MB BChir, DCH, D Obst RCOG. Medical Officer, Christ's Hospital, Horsham (Honorary Editor).

E. J. C. Kendall, MD, MRCP. Formerly Medical Officer, Epsom College.

R. J. R. Moffat, MRCS LRCP, D Obst RCOG, MRCGP. Medical Officer, Whitgift Schools, Croydon.

P. T. Penny, MB BS., MFOM. Medical Officer, Taunton School, Pyrland Hall School and King's College, Taunton; Hon. Medical Adviser, Amateur Swimming Association; Occupational Health Physician, Somerset Health Authority.

H. J. Rose, MB BS, D Obst RCOG. Medical Officer, Downside School.

Isabel G. Smith, MB BS, MRCP, MFCM, DCH, DPH. Medical Adviser, Inner London Education Authority.

J. P. Sparks, MD, FRCP. Medical Officer, Rugby School.

P. de Bec Turtle, OBE, VRD, MA, BM BCh, DPH, FRCGP. Formerly Resident Medical Officer, Haileybury College. *(Died August 1983).*

With the assistance of:

Constance L. Beynon, MB ChB, FRCSE, FRCOG, DPH, JP. Emeritus Consultant in Obstetrics and Gynaecology, Worthing, Southlands, Brighton and Lewes Hospitals; formerly Medical Officer, Roedean School.

J. O. B. Rosedale, MB BS, DCH, D Obst RCOG. Medical Officer, Marlborough College; Medical Officer to the British Everest Expedition, 1972.

CHAPTER 1

RESPONSIBILITIES OF SCHOOL MEDICAL OFFICERS

Introduction

The school doctor should be appointed by the governing body of the school or the local District Health Authority and should be directly responsible to them. The doctor must, however, respect the jurisdiction of the head teacher, who has overall responsibility for the school including the discipline and timetable of the school community.

There are considerable differences in medical organization between maintained and independent schools, and between day and boarding schools. In maintained schools there is a division of responsibility between the school medical officer and the occupational health and environmental health services of the employing authority, but in independent schools the doctor should be responsible for advising on all matters affecting the health of the school. This includes not only the pupils but everybody who is concerned with the working of the school, e.g. teaching and domestic staff, and visitors to the school premises. There is an obligation to provide medical care for any emergency or injury which might occur to members of visiting school teams, for example, and to report details to the patient's own doctor.

The school doctor should carry out medical examinations on pupils as necessary and ensure that regular screening of vision, hearing, height and weight is performed. These matters are dealt with in Chapter 2.

Epidemiological control is important in a school community. The school doctor should see that the pupils are fully immunized in accordance with current DHSS recommendations, and when an infection occurs it is for him to decide when the pupil can be allowed to return to school. Generally, he should have the power to act as the epidemiologist for the prevention and control of infectious diseases. He should, however, realize that the school is part of a larger community for which the District Medical Officer has overall responsibility and with whom he should work in close collaboration. He has a statutory duty to notify certain specified diseases to the Medical Officer for Environmental Health of the local health authority (see Appendix A, p. 182).

When an outbreak of infectious disease occurs it may be appropriate for the school doctor to liaise with the doctor of any other school with which sports fixtures or social events are planned. If care is taken to see that the members of the teams are healthy on the day of the match it should rarely be necessary to cancel fixtures.

The school doctor should actively concern himself with the hygienic condition of the school premises, and, where necessary, call upon the help of an environmental health officer from the local authority. Some doctors like to make annual inspections of the school premises; others keep them under less formal but equally rigorous review. A report should in any case be made at least annually to the governors on the general health of the pupils, the incidence of illness, the level of prophylaxis, and the environmental health of the premises, detailing any alterations or improvements necessary for the promotion of health and well-being of the community.

Administration in maintained schools

The School Health Service was first established in 1907, and the 1973 NHS Reorganization Act transferred responsibility for it from Local Education Authorities to the National Health Service. Since the NHS Reorganisation Act 1981, the service in England and Wales has been the responsibility of the District Health Authorities which manage all community health services for the population within their area. They employ the school medical officers who are on the establishment of the District Medical Officer. In day schools they do not prescribe treatment, but should maintain close contact directly or through the District Medical Officer with the pupils' family doctors. The school nursing service is managed and administered by the Director of Nursing (Community Services). It is good policy for named school doctors and nurses to be responsible for individual schools.

Administration in independent schools

The doctor appointed to an independent boarding school is usually a general practitioner who is contracted both to the Board of Governors of the school and also to the local Family Practitioner Committee for the provision of general medical services. The boarding pupils, and such staff and dependents as elect to do so, register with him under the National Health Service, and he is therefore responsible for providing all general practitioner services during term, and during the holidays if they are resident in the school area. (For those not living locally, any necessary holiday treatment should be obtained under the 'temporary resident' provisions.) The school medical officer is not the doctor of the parents' choice, and to gain their confidence he should do everything possible to build up good relations with the teaching staff, pupils and parents, and liaise closely with the families' general practitioners. The school doctor must be the person responsible for the administration of the services necessary for the nursing of sick or injured pupils and staff.

In a school with day pupils, these pupils are not registered with the school doctor under the National Health Service unless he happens already to be the family doctor. In co-operation with the head teacher, the school doctor should provide for the full medical care of all day pupils during the time they are within the precincts of the school and until they are able to return home under parental care and the supervision of the family doctor.

It is strongly recommended that the school doctor should enter into a contract for services with his employers. A specimen contract is set out in Appendix H, p. 217.

An independent school medical officer has many duties which are outside his National Health Service contractual obligations. They include the following:

(a)   Advising the head and governing body on matters of health.

(b)   Liaison with housemasters, housemistresses and other staff concerning the physical and mental health and fitness of individual pupils.

(c)   The medical supervision of the sanatorium or sick bay, advice on the appointment of nursing staff, and the general direction of their professional duties.

(d)   Periodic medical examination of pupils, including screening for vision, hearing, height and weight.

(e)   Epidemiological surveillance, including maintenance of sickness and injury records additional to clinical notes forming part of the National Health Service records.

(f)   Maintenance of immunization records and arranging immunization programmes to ensure that all pupils are immunized in accordance with current practice recommended by the DHSS, including tetanus, poliomyelitis, measles, BCG and rubella vaccination.

(g)   Liaison with parents: obtaining their informed consent to medical investigations, treatment and immunizations; informing them of procedure in the case of communicable disease occurring at home; and advising them on immunizations and antimalarial drugs for those travelling overseas.

(h)   In collaboration with the head and governing body and, where applicable, the Environmental Health Officer, advising on the hygiene of the school premises.

(i)   Advising on the prevention of accidents and sports injuries, including requirements under the Health and Safety at Work Act.

(j)   Ensuring that pupils receive regular dental inspection either at school or through their parents or guardians.

(k)   Pre-employment medical examinations of teaching and non-teaching staff.

(l)   Incapacity certificates required by the school authorities for employees.

(m)   International Certificates of Vaccination.

(n)   Certificates of freedom from infection, e.g. for CCF camps, travel and employment.

(o)   Reports to university medical officers and certificates of fitness to attend a university or college of further education.

(p)   Certificates required to support claims for benefit from a provident association.

It is not good practice for a doctor to contract to provide less than the full services under items (a) – (j) unless he is satisfied that the items are covered from another source.

Medical services in boarding schools

The sanatorium

All but the smallest of boarding schools should have their own sanatoria, as it is good policy to centralize the provision for sick pupils to allow for supervision by trained staff. Nevertheless, it can never be possible to staff and maintain sufficient beds for epidemics such as influenza. During the postwar era there has been a fall in the bed occupancy of sanatoria and this has resulted in an understandable desire by school authorities to convert sanatorium space to other uses. A detailed review of requirements by MOSA in 1977 concluded that a provision of one bed for every 30 boarders is sufficient for all but the smallest secondary schools. For preparatory schools one bed for every 20 pupils is recommended. Pressure on sanatorium space should not be allowed to bring the numbers of beds below these levels, or to jeopardize the adequate provision of separate nursing facilities for boys and girls in coeducational schools.

A large proportion of beds should be in one-bed units and should be used for observation and isolation. Secondary or cross-infection can be minimized by adequate bed spacing, i.e. not less than 1.8 m between beds in large wards, but it is more surely prevented by isolation in one-bed units. Adequate recreation and dining rooms for convalescents are desirable. There must also be a consulting room and treatment room and a secure, locked room or cupboard for medicines and drugs.

Every school should realize that dormitories will have to be used occasionally as sick rooms, and the head and medical officer should make the necessary plans before the emergency. These may have to be varied with circumstances, but the basic principles should be settled in advance. Architects concerned with new buildings, or with altering old ones, should consider the possibility of having rooms closely associated with the sanatorium which can be used for other purposes.

Government regulations on accommodation for the sick are included in Education (School Premises) Regulations 1981[1], which state in paragraph 19:

'A boarding school shall include, as part of the boarding accommodation:

(a)   one or more sick rooms,

(b) if the school has more than 40 boarding pupils, one or more separate isolation rooms, and

(c) associated facilities by way of baths, washbasins, and water closets, which satisfy the requirements of this Regulation so, however, that in the case of a school attended by both boy and girl boarders some or all of whom have attained the age of 8 years separate sick rooms shall be provided for boys and for girls.

A sick room or isolation room shall be such that:

(a) the floor area is not less than 7.4 m² for each bed therein, and

(b) there is a distance of not less than 1.8 m between any two beds; and, where cubicle accommodation is provided, each cubicle shall have its own window'.

It is not always practicable for preparatory schools to have a sanatorium, and a self-contained sick bay is an acceptable alternative so long as the facilities described above are provided. The matron's living accommodation must be sited so as to allow close supervision of young patients.

Nursing staff

At any time the nurse of a sanatorium should be a State Registered Nurse or a Registered Sick Children's Nurse. Staffing should provide for adequate off-duty and nurses should be paid according to the Whitley Council scale. Many independent schools provide free board and lodging, and therefore arrange their pay scales to provide a net income equivalent to that of a nurse on the Whitley Council scale. It may be necessary to recruit extra temporary nursing staff from an agency at times of epidemics. The school medical officer should be actively involved in the appointment of nursing staff, who should work under his direct control and be responsible to him.

Medical records

A questionnaire should be completed before the entry of each pupil giving the medical history; where there has been significant illness an accompanying letter from the family doctor or consultant is often helpful. The form should be signed by the parent or guardian and sent to the school before the pupil's acceptance, which in rare instances may have to be postponed or refused. The example printed in Appendix B, p. 187, will serve as a guide.

In the case of pupils moving from preparatory to public school, it is of great help to the public school doctor if the pupil is given a card bearing his name, date of birth, NHS number and immunization history with details of any drug sensitivity and current treatment. In the maintained schools this information is given on Form 10M which should be forwarded without delay to the doctor of the new school via the District Medical Officer.

The medical officer has the normal responsibility for keeping records of Form FP7 or 8 under the National Health Service regulations. It is also desirable that special records should be kept for each pupil, incorporating the data on the entrance questionnaire, the findings at the initial examination, and such events of medical importance as may occur during the school life of the pupil. Records must be conspicuously marked with drug sensitivities, and the information should be immediately available to the nursing staff. This can all be incorporated in an A4 file, where all correspondence and hospital reports can be filed, and which is retained after the pupil has left. The alternative is a school medical record card which can be placed in the pupil's FP5 or 6 on leaving school. Whatever method is used it is important that a summary is placed in the NHS card envelope, and a rubber stamp worded as follows on the FP7 or 8 can be useful:

> 'This patient was a pupil at ....school from ....to .... Only major items (taken from fuller notes) are entered below. If further details are wanted, please write to the Medical Officer, ...'

The school doctor has a responsibility to inform teachers of medical problems which may affect the educational progress and fitness for physical activity of the pupils. The administrative details are a matter for the individual, but may take the form of a list displayed in the teaching staff common room, which must be periodically brought up to date. This should include such obvious medical disorders as epilepsy, diabetes and bleeding diatheses, as well as defects of hearing and vision. In maintained schools essential information including immunization history has to be given to the head teacher in a special record to be held in the child's education file, and it is the doctor's responsibility to keep these records up to date.

Medical regulations

Medical regulations should be formulated and circulated so that parents know what the school's requirements are. The need for quarantine and isolation after infectious diseases has now almost disappeared in the case of diseases commonly acquired in the United Kingdom, but in contrast greater vigilance is needed in respect of pupils returning from abroad, to prevent the spread of enteric and exotic infection.

A clear statement should be obtained from the parent about medical insurance: whether the family subscribes to a provident association and prefers private treatment from consultants, and whether they wish to participate in an accident insurance scheme.

A specimen form of advice to parents is included in Appendix B, p. 192.

Information to parents regarding current illness

In all cases of illness among pupils, the parents or guardians should be informed and should be supplied with progress reports as necessary. Whether this is done in the case of routine illness by the head, housemaster or housemistress, or by the doctor or sister in charge of the sanatorium, must be a matter for local arrangement. Nevertheless, the school doctor will be well advised to acquaint parents direct (by telephone if possible) in the case of accident or severe illness.

Whenever possible, and for all 'cold' surgery, the hospital authority for operation or anaesthetic for all children under the age of 16 should be signed by the parent or legal guardian. When it is not possible to contact the parents in an emergency, it is for the doctor in charge of the case to do whatever he thinks necessary in the best interests of the patient. In practice, it is usually helpful for the head teacher or deputy acting *in loco parentis* to sign the consent form.

Section 8 of the Family Law Reform Act 1969 provides that the consent to medical, surgical and dental treatment of a minor who has attained the age of 16 years shall be effective consent. Over this age, therefore, the hospital consent form should be signed by the pupil although the parents or guardian should be kept informed.

Schools have a responsibility for letting parents know when children have been exposed to infection at school and may develop the disease during the holidays. Dates should be given to include the appropriate incubation period. This is of particular importance in the case of rubella, when pupils incubating the disease may come into contact with women in the first trimester of pregnancy.

School closure

Even in the days when poliomyelitis was common, MOSA argued forcefully against the practice of school closure as a preventive measure. In today's conditions it is hard to envisage any situation which would justify it, and it should certainly not be contemplated without reference to the Medical Officer for Environmental Health.

Advisory responsibilities of the school doctor

There are many areas in which the school doctor's influence should be felt, and most of them will form the subject matter of the ensuing chapters. Others are more suitably introduced here.

Diet

School catering is increasingly managed by professionally qualified staff. The school meals service is centrally controlled and subject to financial constraint by the local education authorities, and the individual school doctor can have little influence on it. In independent schools his responsibilities are greater and he should be concerned to see that the diet is nutritionally balanced, sufficiently varied, attractively served and adequate for the energy needs of the growing child. A guide to the nutritional requirements of different age groups can be found in the 1979 Report of the DHSS Committee on Medical Aspects of Food Policy[2]. The doctor should use his influence to encourage a diet high in fibre and low in animal fat and to discourage excessive intake of foods and drinks which lead to caries. In practice this means the encouragement of bran-containing breakfast cereals, wholemeal bread and fresh fruit, with some degree of control on the consumption of sweets and sucrose-rich drinks; liaison with the tuck-shop management over hours of opening and types of food sold can be helpful in this respect. The doctor should take an interest in the type of cooking oil used in the kitchens, in order to encourage the use of polyunsaturated fats such as corn oil rather than cheaper substitutes.

Obesity is a common condition in growing children and the school doctor should liaise with the catering staff on the provision of a satisfactory low-calorie diet. He should also advise about the diet of diabetic pupils and others with special dietary needs.

Rest and exercise

Throughout its history, MOSA has been concerned to prevent the erosion by boarding schools of the hours of sleep needed by pupils. Present knowledge does not permit us to lay down dogmatic rules, but there is no doubt that most schools need the restraining influence of the medical officer on some aspects of the school timetable. A recent study of sleep behaviour[3] which measured the actual duration of sleep of a large group of children of various ages confirmed that sleep needs differ considerably among children of the same age, so that one cannot specify how many hours of sleep they ought to have at a certain age. However, the mean duration of sleep, day and night, found in this study was greater than that provided by some boarding school timetables, and it is the most useful guide we have: 11 hours at 7 years, 10 hours at 11 years, and 9 hours at 15 years.

It is also difficult to be dogmatic about the interval necessary between meals and vigorous exercise, although there can be no doubt that such an interval is necessary. Most would agree that it should be at least half an hour.

Health education

Despite a plethora of official publications, the position of health education in the curriculum is often a tenuous one. The interested school doctor can make a valuable contribution, and may be the only person in a school to press for its proper emphasis. When he has a gift for teaching, and can spare the time, he may take an active place in the teaching team. First aid is the subject most likely to fall to his lot, and no opportunity should be lost to teach the basic skill of mouth-to-mouth resuscitation. Every school should possess teaching aids such as the 'Resusci-Andy' and 'Resusci-Anne' manikins for this purpose.

The history, range, and continuing uncertainties of health education are comprehensively covered in the Department of Education and Science book *Health Education in Schools*[4], which is commended to the interested reader. Further comments on drug and sex education are to be found in Chapter 4 (p. 71).

The Health Education Council provides health education material and has a Resources Centre which provides up-to-date publications and teaching aids.

Address

The Health Education Council, 78 New Oxford Street, London WC1A 1AH.

Dental supervision

The school doctor should be concerned with the provision of good dental care. In maintained schools the Health Authority is obliged to arrange for all children to be dentally examined at intervals by the Community Dental Service, and the medical officer can refer pupils to the school dental officer. In independent schools, it is possible for children to miss this essential service unless the medical officer takes active steps to see that there is a reliable routine by which children see a dentist in the school holidays if there is no provision at school. The National Health Service regulations are specifically framed to enable boarding school children to attend for inspections three times a year. An alternative solution is for boarding schools to arrange for a dental surgeon to attend regularly to carry out inspections and treatment in termtime of all pupils except those whose parents wish them to remain under the care of a dentist at home. The increasing use of mouthguards in sport and of orthodontic treatment, with its need for frequent adjustment of appliances, are other factors in favour of such an arrangement. The dental surgeon attending a school should also make a contribution to individual and group health education on the preventive aspects of oral hygiene, including the care of the teeth, discouragement of caries-inducing diet and the prevention of sports injury through mouthguards (see also p. 108).

Counselling

The school doctor should be in a good position to co-ordinate the various agencies which are available for counselling, and to act as a link between teaching staff, social services and the school psychological service. The doctor may or may not undertake individual counselling, according to his own inclinations and training and the strength of the non-medical counselling in the school. His responsibilities are possibly greater in independent schools which may not have easy access to the maintained schools' channels of referral to the school psychological service; maintained school doctors can also assist the teaching staff in recognizing and referring children with emotional and psychiatric problems. Some independent schools have found it valuable to retain the services of a psychiatrist with an interest in child and adolescent emotional disorders, both for individual referrals and to help the staff of the school to develop their counselling skills[5].

Remuneration

Maintained schools and Local Authority establishments

Medical Officers in the School Health Service are paid a salary on the national scale. Rates for establishments maintained by Local Authorities are published annually, but apply to a diminishing number of doctors.

Independent schools

From the beginning of the National Health Service in 1948 it was established that medical officers of independent schools would normally accept the pupils as patients on their NHS list, and receive in addition to their NHS remuneration a fee from the school for duties lying outside the NHS.

MOSA and the BMA recommend that the basis of payment should be a *per capita* fee and it is a common practice in many fee-paying schools for these charges to be passed on to the parents by the school authorities. It must be emphasized that no fee can be claimed for any duty which is covered by the National Health Service Act, 1946. The duties which are covered by the fee are listed on pp. 3–4. Doctors are entitled to charge individual fees for items (k) – (p), but these might well be waived by the medical officer who is in receipt of the recommended capitation fee. The exact fee is a matter for negotiation between the medical officer and the school, who are both advised to enter into a contract which provides for an annual salary review (See Appendix H, p. 217). Guidance on the amount of the capitation fee to be negotiated is provided annually by MOSA and the BMA. The MOSA recommended rate is circulated to members and the BMA recommendation is included in Section VI of the Fees section of its Handbook. In the past the recommendation was agreed jointly by MOSA and the BMA, but since 1979 the two organisations have been unable to reach agreement and have therefore published different recommendations, the BMA rate being the higher of the two.

References

1. Statutory instrument No. 909 (1981). *The Education (School Premises) Regulations 1981*. (London: HMSO)
2. Department of Health and Social Security (1979). *Recommended daily amounts of food energy and nutrients for groups of people in the United Kingdom*. Report on Health and Social Subjects 15. (London: HMSO)

3. Klackenberg, G. (1982). Sleep behaviour studied longitudinally. *Acta Paediatr. Scand.*, 71, 501

4. Department of Education and Science (1977). *Health Education in Schools*. (London: HMSO)

5. Cox, M. and Hoskins, T. (1973). Collaboration between psychiatrist and medical officer in a boys' boarding school. *Practitioner*, 210, 209

CHAPTER 2

PREVENTIVE MEDICINE IN SCHOOLS

General hygiene

The school doctor should take an interest in the facilities and hygiene of the school as these are important factors in the health and safety of the community. He should be available to advise the authorities on these matters and should be conversant with the standards laid down by the Department of Education and Science. Tactful investigation of the circumstances of illness and injury may reveal shortcomings which might be rectified by improved conditions or removal of hazards.

The school doctor should establish a useful contact with his District Health Authority colleagues. The Environmental Health Officer is always available to give advice and has a statutory right to inspect all institutional catering facilities.

School premises

Standards are laid down in the Education (School Premises) Regulations 1981[1], of which the main provisions are summarized in Appendix C, p. 194.

Swimming pools

Treatment and quality of swimming pool water

There is no obvious alternative to chlorine as a water disinfectant, but chlorine gas has been phased out and an alternative source of chlorine has to be used. Whichever chlorine donor is decided upon, the active constituent is hypochlorous acid, which is measured in a swimming pool as the *free chlorine residual*. This kills micro-organisms, and also reacts with bather contaminants, mainly urea and creatinine, to produce various irritants to mucous membranes. Some of these are volatile and produce the characteristic swimming pool odour. They also cause irritation of the eyes and respiratory system. All these irritant substances are contained in the *combined chlorine residual*. To minimize irritation this should be kept as low as possible, and not allowed to rise above 1 part per million. With a high bathing load, and therefore heavy bather contamination, the combined chlorine residual should be kept low by frequent back-washing of the filters to dilute the pool water. Alternatively, additional fresh water may be added to the pool. Chlorine itself does not cause eye and respiratory irritation in the absence of bather contaminants: a free chlorine residual high enough to bleach hair and costumes is comfortable for swimming in the absence of contamination.

A well-maintained pool should be clear and colourless, but the pool and its surrounds may give the water a blue appearance. It should not be obviously cloudy, and it should be possible to see clearly through 40 feet of water, not only for aesthetic reasons but also to minimize the risk of undetected drowning accidents. Green colouration which is thought to be due to algae should be treated with five times the usual level of free chlorine residual; the filters should be kept running 24 hours a day and the high chlorine left to reduce before bathing is resumed.

Eye irritation

Any liquid which is not isotonic causes some eye irritation, but the main cause is the substances in the combined chlorine residual. Other chemicals can worsen eye irritation; these include algicides, which should preferably be avoided, and other salts which may be used to correct pH. Unphysiological pH can also affect the eyes. There is no evidence that eye irritation is any less with non-chlorine-based disinfectants, despite advertising to the contrary.

Swimming pool rash and swimmer's ear

The predisposing and causative factors of these conditions are very similar. They include wetting, wetting/drying cycles, degreasing and dewaxing by the disinfectant, infection (usually with some serotypes of *Pseudomonas aeruginosa)*, chemical irritation and acclimatization. In subjects who swim less than once a day, otitis externa should affect less than 1% of a large sample at any time, unless a failure of disinfection has allowed bacteria to build up in the pool. If more than 10% are affected by otitis externa, infection of the pool is almost certain. When infection begins to build up in a pool, swimmers are affected first by otitis externa.

Swimming pool body rash occurs only with very heavy bacterial contamination of the pool, or because of an individual's susceptibility to the disinfectant. Rashes have been reported associated with bromine disinfectants[2] but are very rare with chlorine disinfectants.

Choice of disinfectant

Technical details of the choice of swimming pool disinfectant and methods of working for pool staff are given in Appendix D, p. 197.

Swimming pool safety

This is dealt with in Chapter 8, p. 116.

Water and food hygiene

Water supply

Nearly all schools are supplied from the mains water supply of the local water authority which is responsible for the purity of the supply. In the rare cases where schools have their own water supply, the medical officer will need to enlist the help of the Environmental Health Officer to ensure that it is regularly tested and, where appropriate, chlorinated. It is also important to ensure that plumbo-solvency and pH are satisfactory. In some older school premises a check should be made for lead-lined storage tanks and lead pipes.

Milk supply

It is essential that all milk supplied to schools should be pasteurized. Domestic methods of heat treatment are unreliable and home-produced milk is best disposed of to the Milk Marketing Board, which carries out bulk pasteurization. Milk-borne outbreaks of salmonellosis and campylobacter enteritis appear to be increasing[3] even though they can be completely prevented by adequate pasteurization. In Scotland it has been illegal to supply unpasteurized milk since 1983.

Kitchen hygiene

School kitchens come within the provisions of the Food Hygiene (General) Regulations 1970[4]. The Environmental Health Officer has a responsibility for inspection and maintenance of satisfactory standards. The school doctor should not only be conversant with the Regulations, but should visit kitchens and dining rooms and be prepared to advise catering staff when necessary.

Adequate sanitary facilities, including washbasins with hot water, soap and disposable paper towels or hot air hand driers must be provided for catering staff, and notices displayed near lavatories advising users to wash their hands after using them. A first aid box including waterproof dressings must be provided, and its supplies frequently inspected and replenished. Adequate ventilation and lighting are important for the efficient working of kitchen staff. Kitchen waste should be removed from the kitchen. Refuse bins, preferably galvanized, with lids, or disposable paper sacks should be sited in a dry area outside the kitchen. Some authorities will hire out large refuse containers for institutional use.

Separate stores should be provided for dry goods and for prepared foods. Adequate refrigeration is essential. The time between cooking and eating all cooked moist dishes, especially those containing meat, should be as short as possible, unless provision is made for storage at a temperature above 145°F (62.7°C) or in the cold. The Food Hygiene Regulations require hot food to be kept at a temperature of not less than 145°F (62.7°C) and food to be eaten cold below 50°F (10°C). Large masses of food are more difficult to heat and slower to cool, hence cuts of meat should be limited in size to 6 lb or less. Meat should be prepared and cooked on the day it is to be eaten; re-heating should be discouraged and it should never be left overnight in a warm kitchen. Meat to be eaten cold should be cooled rapidly, preferably in a cold room with fan, and transferred to the refrigerator within 1½ hours of cooking. The temperature of refrigerators should be checked to ensure that a temperature of 34–38°F (1–4°C) is being maintained.

In a review of over 1000 outbreaks of food poisoning and salmonellosis, the Food Hygiene Laboratory at Colindale found that in more than 60% of the outbreaks the food had been prepared over half a day before it was consumed[5]. The report continued, 'This alone would not necessarily cause food poisoning but in combination with inadequate cooling and storage it becomes an extremely important factor. The other main factors were storage at ambient temperature (39.6%), inadequate cooling (31.9%), inadequate reheating (28.5%) and the use of contaminated processed food (19.1%). The latter included foods such as meats and poultry, pies and take away meals prepared in premises other than those in which the final dish was consumed, but not canned foods'. The report notes that infected food handlers did not play a significant role in causation except in *Staph. aureus* food poisoning.

The school doctor should be available to advise on the health of kitchen staff. Superficial cuts must be carefully covered and supervised, and in the event of skin sepsis and gastrointestinal infection food handlers must be excluded from work until symptomatically recovered.

Health of the staff

School doctors are often asked to advise whether an applicant for a teaching, administrative or domestic post is medically fit to be employed. In doing so he cannot reveal his reasons without the applicant's permission. Before an important post is filled it is advisable for the school doctor to obtain a confidential medical report from the applicant's general practitioner and to examine the applicant before declaring him fit for employment.

DES regulations[6] state that a chest X-ray is compulsory for all teachers on first entry to the profession. Many authorities consider that this minimum requirement is insufficient in the light of continuing instances of pulmonary tuberculosis in schools, and it is advisable to require evidence of a satisfactory chest X-ray within the past one or two years.

Particular vigilance is required in the case of part-time as well as full-time domestic staff, who may be immigrants with a risk of importing tuberculosis and other diseases. They may also be employed by catering contractors whose own standard of surveillance may not be as high as that of the school to whom they are contracted.

Women teachers should be advised about protection against rubella (see p. 42).

Disinfection

Heat and ionizing irradiation are the most effective methods of killing micro-organisms, and wherever possible one or other of these methods should be used in preference to chemical disinfectants. Use should be made of the Central Sterile Supply of Dressing and Instruments provided by hospitals, laboratories and local authorities. Sterile disposable syringes and needles should be used. Where an autoclave is installed the manufacturer's instructions should be followed and Browne's tubes should be incorporated in dressings as a check on the efficiency of sterilization.

New disinfectants are constantly introduced to the market, making it difficult to know which are effective and economical for any particular purpose. Disinfection is not a substitute for cleanliness. Unless proper cleaning methods are followed the disinfection may be hampered. The use of disinfectants is not a cover for inefficient work.

Broadly, disinfectants can be grouped under five headings:

(a) *Phenols, cresols, etc.,* including black and white fluids, Lysol, Jeyes Fluid, Izal and Stericol.

(b) *Chlorine-substituted phenols,* including the chloroxylenols and chlorhexidines (Chloroxylenol solution, Dettol, Hibitane, etc.), and combinations of these with other preparations, such as chlorhexidine and cetrimide (Savlon).

(c) *Halogen compounds,* including hypochlorites, Eusol, Dakin's solution, Chloros, Milton, etc., and combinations of these with other preparations such as hypochlorite and detergent (Diton), iodine and povidone-iodine (Betadine).

(d) *Quaternary ammonium compounds,* including cetrimide (Cetavlon) and benzalkonium (Roccal).

(e) *Miscellaneous chemicals,* including acridine and its derivatives, hexachlorophane (Cidal), formaldehyde, alcohol, mercury compounds, hydrogen peroxide, certain dyes, etc.

The phenols and cresols retain their germicidal efficiency remarkably well in the presence of organic matter, but it falls off rapidly with increasing dilution. They are useful general purpose disinfectants. The value of chloroxylenols is reduced in the presence of blood or serum. Hypochlorites generally are most useful disinfectants, but solutions, especially when diluted, deteriorate quickly in the presence of organic matter or when exposed to sunlight. The quaternary ammonium compounds possess high surface activity with excellent detergent properties and make good skin disinfectants, but their bactericidal action is reduced or even removed by soap. Cetrimide and allied compounds are used extensively; containers may become contaminated with *Pseudomonas,* and cork closures should be avoided.

Swabs impregnated with isopropyl alcohol and chlorhexidine are manufactured for skin cleansing prior to injection, but there is no evidence that they are necessary if the skin is socially clean[7].

The following methods are recommended for general use in school sanatoria.

Baths and basins

Baths and basins should be thoroughly cleaned after use with a detergent and hypochlorite.

Bath mats

It is difficult even to ensure cleanliness of the bath mats in common use. Bath mats, like duckboards in swimming baths and showers, should be discarded.

Bed linen

Ordinarily the usual laundering process is adequate for sheets and pillow cases.

Bedpans, bottles and chamber-pots

Unless disposable, these should be efficiently cleaned after use and, where necessary, they should also be disinfected. Where heat disinfection is impracticable bedpans, etc. should be immersed after cleaning in Stericol 1% for 30 minutes in receptacles kept for this purpose alone. Plastic bedpans are recommended.

Bedsteads

Washing with soap or detergent and hot water is adequate.

Blankets

Heat disinfection damages woollen blankets in time and shortens their useful life. Consideration should be given to their replacement in sanatoria by cellular blankets of terylene, nylon or cotton which can be boiled.

Crockery and cutlery

All crockery and cutlery should be of a kind which can be boiled without coming to harm. Where possible it should be washed in the first section of a double sink and then kept for at least two minutes in the sterilizing section at a temperature of not less than 180°F (82°C). Where sterilizing sinks have not been installed crockery should be thoroughly washed in detergent and hot water. When there is risk of the spread of intestinal infection each patient should have his own crockery, which should be boiled after washing.

Automatic dishwashers should be of a type which not only cleans but also sterilizes.

Tea towels and dishcloths are dealt with in the section on towels.

Drains and gullies

These should be kept clean and free from obstruction. If an offensive smell persists the Environmental Health Officer should be consulted. Do not waste money by pouring disinfectants down the drain.

Dressings

Soiled dressings should be put in disposable containers and placed in a pedal-operated bin before being disposed of in a gas-fired incinerator.

Face masks

Disposable face masks should be used.

Floors

Floors in sanatoria should be washable, non-absorbent and not slippery. Good quality linoleum is satisfactory. Wooden floors should be treated to reduce the amount of dust. Spindle oil was used for some years but is largely replaced now by special 'seals' which give a non-slip surface which can easily be kept clean. The use of disinfectants in the solution used for cleaning floors is unnecessary.

Handkerchiefs

It is preferable to use disposable paper handkerchiefs which should be placed after use in disposable containers and burned. If this is impracticable bedside bowls should be provided in which to keep handkerchiefs. The handkerchiefs should be soaked overnight in chloroxylenol (1:80) before being laundered.

Instruments

When not disposable, these should be sterilized by the local central sterile supply service. Boxes must be provided for disposable needles and other sharp objects to avoid the risk of pricking anybody who handles them before incineration.

Mattresses

Where necessary, ordinary mattresses can be sterilized by steam, but this does reduce their useful (and comfortable) life. This disadvantage can be avoided by the use of plastic mattress covers which can be cleaned. Rubber mattresses can be swabbed with white fluid (1:40) and then washed with soap and water.

Nail-brushes

Only nylon and plastic brushes should be used in sanatoria. Between use the nail-brushes can stand in a solution of chloroxylenol (1:80).

Spatulas

Wooden spatulas should be used and discarded after using once. If, for any reason, other kinds of spatula have to be used, they should be sterilized by boiling.

Sputum mugs

These should be boiled for ten minutes after emptying. A little white fluid (1:20) should be placed in the mug before it is used. Disposable mugs or linings can be used.

Syringes

Sterile disposable syringes should be used. If this is not possible syringes should be sterilized by the local central sterile supply service.

Towels

Hand towels and bath towels should be individually supplied. When not in use they should be hung where they do not touch other towels.

Roller towels and cabinet-type pull-down towels should be replaced by good quality paper towels in an efficient dispensing fitment, and this can be supplemented by hot-air hand driers.

As a general rule the use of tea towels and dishcloths should be avoided by the installation of sterilizing sinks. Where tea towels must be used they should be boiled frequently.

Urinals

The smell sometimes arising from urinals can be dispelled when the deposit and scale on the urinals are removed. The frequent use of lavatory cleanser followed by washing down with hot water is recommended for this purpose. If the smell persists the assistance of the local Environmental Health Officer should be sought.

Walls

Walls should be washed when necessary with soap or detergent and water if they are suitable for such treatment. The walls of sanatoria should be painted to provide a washable surface; dust-holding ledges such as picture rails should be removed. Cresol disinfectants should not be used for washing walls as they have paint-removing qualities.

Water closets and sluices

These should be designed so that they can easily be cleaned; ideally, the wall-hanging type should be fitted. The use of wooden seats is undesirable as they are porous and easily become fissured: plastic, open-ended seats are much better. Lavatory cleanser is recommended for cleaning the pan. It is wasteful to pour disinfectants into the pan.

For cleaning the floor, door handles, chain pulls, etc. ordinary domestic cleaning is adequate in normal times, but these should be wiped with white fluid (1:40) when intestinal infections are present.

Terminal disinfection

Terminal disinfection, after the patient has been removed or ceased to be a source of infection, is no longer practised. Terminal cleaning suffices along with airing and sunning of rooms, furniture and bedding. It is required only for diseases spread by indirect contact. Cleaning involves scrubbing with hot water and detergent all surfaces where organic matter may have accumulated.

Isolation

The need for isolation of patients in school practice has greatly diminished in recent years. The dangerous infectious diseases are rare and should be transferred to an isolation hospital as soon as the diagnosis becomes likely, but there is seldom any need for strict isolation for the common communicable diseases, as their spread is little affected by it. Single rooms should be used for nursing patients with extensive skin sepsis, streptococcal throat infections in the first 24 hours of treatment, meningitis, salmonella infections, dysentery, diarrhoea of unknown cause, and viral hepatitis.

Scrupulous personal hygiene and hand-washing by attendants are essential but schools seldom have sufficient staff to make barrier nursing practicable. The only common exception is viral hepatitis, which is spread by blood, faeces and urine, and the greatest care should be taken to prevent transmission, especially when hepatitis-B has not been excluded. Staff with cuts and abrasions should not attend hepatitis patients. Blood should only be taken by doctors wearing gloves and taking special precautions to avoid contact with blood. The specimen must be sent to the laboratory in a sealed plastic bag labelled 'High risk specimen', and the request form boldly marked 'Hepatitis'. Spilled blood, faeces or urine should be covered with hypochlorite disinfectant before being mopped up. If anyone is pricked with a needle or other sharp instrument which has been used on a patient with hepatitis, the skin should be immediately washed and the incident reported to the doctor. Hepatitis-specific immunoglobulin should be given if available.

In patients with enteric infections and hepatitis, bedpans and urinals, if used, must be washed and disinfected after each use or must be disposable; hands must be thoroughly washed after dealing with them, and by the patient after every bowel action and urination. Dressings, disposable syringes, and other burnable items are put into small paper bags in the patient's room, and needles put into 'sharps' boxes and then incinerated.

For routine cleaning of isolation rooms normal domestic methods without disinfectant are used, but mops and cleaning cloths are rinsed daily in phenolic disinfectant.

Quarantine

Quarantine was the time-honoured method of preventing the spread of infectious disease from ships. The name derives from the 40 day period during which a quarantined ship was kept out of port. It was then adopted for the exclusion of contacts from school, a practice that was often rigorously applied until Simey broke with tradition at Rugby School in 1927. Statistical confirmation that he was correct was subsequently provided by his successor, Smith[8]. Unfortunately, it took a little time for the tradition to be given up in many schools.

There is no justification for excluding contacts of communicable disease from school, except in the case of three diseases which are now rare in Europe: diphtheria, typhoid and poliomyelitis. Prolonged exclusion is seldom justifiable even for these diseases, and the Medical Officer for Environmental Health should always be consulted. It is also advisable to exclude nursery and primary school children whose siblings have bacillary dysentery.

School medical examinations

School medical examinations have been a vital component of preventive medicine ever since their introduction as a compulsory measure by the Education Act of 1907. Their function has been reassessed at intervals since that time. It is now generally held that the essential components of a child's routine medical examination are developmental screening in the early years, a medical examination at 5 years, during the first year at primary school, and a further examination at some time before leaving school. Court[9] recommended that 'every boy or girl at about the age of 13 should have a private interview with the school doctor': in the independent sector this may conveniently be on entry to public school. It is not now thought that repeated medical examinations are of enough value as a routine measure to justify the expenditure of time and resources, but the 5-year-old medical examination should bring to light those children in whom selective follow-up is necessary. Regular screening of vision, hearing, height and weight are necessary throughout school life. Although there has been recent discussion on blood pressure screening, there is not sufficient evidence that its benefits would outweigh the disadvantages: apart from the high cost of a universal screening programme, a great deal of anxiety would be caused to parents and children whose blood pressure may be labile but not require treatment. A single measurement at the 13-year-old medical would identify those in whom follow-up might be indicated.

Developmental screening

Developmental screening should start in infancy, and although the later examinations may overlap with the nursery school years, the details are not within the scope of this Handbook. They may be found in many standard works such as Illingworth's[10].

The school entrant examination

Starting school is an important milestone in the life of every child and the entrant medical examination is the most important examination during school life. It is best conducted during the second term, after the child has had a chance to settle into school. The parents and teacher should participate in the discussions, and the examination should be unhurried. Fifteen minutes should be allowed for each child and the examination should include assessment of the child's physical, emotional, intellectual and social development.

The examination should be preceded, on the previous day or earlier, by screening tests which can be carried out in most cases by the school nurse. In maintained schools the results of the screening tests and examinations are entered, with the social and medical history, on Form 10M. The screening tests are as follows.

Height and weight

Reference to Tanner and Whitehouse charts (see Appendix E) will identify those children falling outside the normal range for their age, and these will require scrutiny. Obesity is a common finding, and the doctor should take the opportunity to give advice to parents and child; it may be necessary to request low calorie meals from the

school. Much more rarely, children with growth hormone deficiency and hypothyroidism are detected by routine measurement at
the school entrance examination; there is then still time for treatment to be effective[11].

Hearing

The identification of children with any degree of hearing loss is
essential, because children who have even a mild degree of hearing
loss will be at a considerable disadvantage educationally if the
condition is not diagnosed. All children at school entry should have
their hearing screened by pure tone audiometry. Conditions for
carrying out the tests often leave much to be desired and vigilance is
necessary to ensure that children with hearing loss are not missed,
and that appropriate action is taken and followed through in all
cases of doubt.

Vision

The best test of visual acuity for entrants and nursery children is the
Gardiner–Sheridan Stycar test. Alternatively Snellen charts may be
used. Colour vision is also tested, using the Guy's Test for Colour
Vision or a modification of the Ishihara Test of Colour Vision.
    It has been shown that, because of the use of coloured materials in
the teaching of infants, a child with defective colour vision is apprec-
iably disadvantaged in his early school life. If a child is found to have
defective colour vision the teachers should be told and the difficulties which are likely to arise explained to them. The parents should,
of course, also be advised of the problem. A specimen information
sheet on defective colour vision is given in Appendix F (p. 211).

Urine

Form 10M makes no specific mention of urine tests, presumably
because of the practical difficulties of collecting and testing specimens in the primary school environment. This must result in delay
in diagnosis of some cases of diabetes and pyelonephritis, which
some school doctors will wish to remedy. At the very least, a urine
test should be part of the 13-year-old medical examination.

Screening for haemoglobinopathies

The trait or disease of sickle cell anaemia and other haemoglobinopathies may be carried by Negro and coloured children. They are normally screened at birth if born in the United Kingdom. School medical examinations afford an opportunity to identify those born overseas who have not been screened. A haemoglobin estimation will identify children requiring further investigation.

With the results of the screening tests to hand, and if possible a brief medical history obtained in advance from the parent by means of a questionnaire, the doctor is ready to carry out the medical examination. Parents are entitled by law to be present in maintained schools, and should be encouraged to attend, but education authorities have a duty to examine children unless the parent objects, and examinations should proceed even in the absence of a parent. Where possible, the doctor obtains an obstetric and perinatal history from the mother and also obtains information from the clinic notes. He should ask about past illnesses, for example otitis media, fits or habit disorders such as enuresis, and the mother can discuss any worries she may have about her child. During the early stages of each interview the doctor will have noted the general appearance of the children, their gait, the presence of any asymmetry, and whether their behaviour is appropriate to their age and situation. As they draw a picture observation should be made about their laterality and pencil grasp. A request to copy a square (5-year level) or a circle (3-year level) is a quick test to indicate developmental retardation, and other tests can be added if necessary. Children will often explain what they have drawn and so give the doctor an opportunity to hear them speak. A full physical examination is required, but undressing should not be attempted until the end of the interview when children are ready to accept the removal of their clothes, including shoes and socks. The majority will speak during the interview, but if they do not, the doctor should assess their speech and articulation by asking them to repeat sentences or name pictures in a simple picture book. Abnormalities of speech in schoolchildren are most commonly found among the infants, and it is important to be certain that their hearing is normal before speech therapy is recommended.

Children who have been found on screening to have visual defects should be examined for abnormalities such as inequality of the pupils or nystagmus, and should be tested for squint using the corneal light reflex and the cover test. Children who have squints or other ocular pathology or whose visual acuity is defective should be referred for a consultant ophthalmological opinion. Particular attention should be paid to children found to have defective hearing: they should be referred to a consultant audiologist and followed up.

The general examination is best started with the child standing, as it is convenient for examining the head, ears, nose, throat and chest. In this position many trivial benign heart sounds are inaudible: fuller examination with the child lying or after exercise can be carried out if necessary to elucidate possible abnormalities. The presence of the femoral pulses should be confirmed to exclude coarctation of the aorta. At the same time the hernial orifices and genitalia can be examined. Boys with undescended, as opposed to retractile, testes should be referred for a surgical opinion as early as possible. The forward bending test as a screening for scoliosis can easily be carried out by the doctor, if it has not been delegated to the nurse with other screening procedures. There is a tendency for school doctors to overdiagnose minor orthopaedic conditions for which no treatment is necessary. Flat feet do not need treatment except in cases of extreme eversion or pain, and only severe degrees of knock knee and bowed tibiae require referral.

Subsequent examinations

The school entrant examination provides a profile of each child. Children who show developmental delay should be reviewed regularly by the school doctor, and also those in whom there is a physical condition likely to result in a continuing abnormality. The physical conditions needing supervision include visual or hearing defects, asthma, epilepsy, congenital abnormalities, and physical handicap. The possible adverse effects of any defect on a child's educational progress should be discussed by the doctor and teacher, and ways of minimizing these effects considered.

It is essential that screening of hearing and vision should be repeated at intervals. Audiometry should be carried out again at about 8 years, as secretory otitis media may cause undetected hearing impairment affecting a child's education. Follow-up must be at frequent intervals in all cases of doubt. Visual acuity should be tested at least biennially during school life because of the common onset of myopia around puberty.

Although weighing and measuring of children is no longer routine practice in many schools, there is much to be said for it at a time when both obesity and anorexia nervosa are so common. The highest incidence of anorexia nervosa is among girls in independent schools, and it may be most readily detected if there is a regular routine of weighing pupils. In any case, those children falling out-side the 3 and 97 centiles on Tanner's charts should have their heights and weights regularly measured and charted.

Subsequent medical examinations of primary school children are performed on a selective basis. Questionnaires may be completed by the parents and returned to the school, and a decision is made to call the children up for examination after consultation between the school doctor and the teaching staff. Examination after transfer to secondary school is advisable, particularly as this may coincide with the onset of puberty and a period of rapid growth.

The parents and teachers should be encouraged to bring to the doctor's attention emotional or behavioural problems that their children show. If there is insufficient time to deal adequately with a particular child during the medical examination, the doctor should arrange either another visit to the school or an appointment for the child to be seen as a special case in a clinic. Children who are making poor educational progress should be seen by an educational psychologist, and if emotional or behaviour factors are considered to need help, referral to the child and adolescent psychiatric service is advisable.

The school leaver examination

This should be carried out at some time between 13 years and leaving school. The school leaver's fitness for all types of work should be assessed and Form Y9 completed for any pupil whose choice of employment should be restricted for health reasons, including all those with defective colour vision. Copies of the form are sent to Careers Officers and the Employment Medical Adviser. For pupils with severe handicaps, Form Y10 may be appropriate: it is used for children in special schools and those who may qualify for registration as a disabled person.

School medical examinations in independent schools

All the foregoing principles apply to independent as well as main-tained schools. Regrettably, not all independent schools arrange for medical examination and screening of their pupils, and there is no statutory obligation upon them to do so. It is therefore doubly important for the doctor of an independent school to examine pupils entering the school, having obtained as full a history as possible. Briscoe[12] has described the advantages in terms of pupil–doctor–parent relationships as well as the purely medical benefit of a thorough entrance medical examination on public school entry. Special examinations are often required for those embarking on hazardous sports or adventure training, and a suitably high standard of physical and psychological fitness must be looked for.`

Most independent schools make use of the following procedures to make up the confidential medical record of each individual:

(a) A questionnaire concerning details of the family history, previous health and immunization history. A specimen is printed in Appendix B, p. 187.

(b) Screening tests to assess visual acuity, colour vision, hearing, height and weight, urine test, tuberculin test, and where necessary, chest X-ray.

(c) The physical examination by the school doctor, who should be in possession of the above information.

In addition to these, but not necessarily as part of the medical procedure, schools may request the following which are of value to the doctor in broadening his knowledge of the pupil:

(d) A report from the child's school, concerning learning or perceptual difficulties and emotional problems.

(e) Special examinations, such as psychometric testing.

References

1. Statutory Instrument No. 909 (1981). *The Education (School Premises) Regulations 1981*. (London: HMSO)
2. Rycroft, R. J. G. and Penny, P. T. (1983). Dermatoses associated with brominated swimming pools. *Br. Med. J.*, 287, 462
3. Galbraith, N. S., Forbes, P. and Clifford, C. (1982). Communicable diseases associated with milk and dairy products in England and Wales 1951–80. *Br. Med. J.*, 284, 1761
4. Statutory Instrument No. 1172 (1970). *The Food Hygiene (General) Regulations 1970*. (London: HMSO)
5. Roberts, D. (1982). Factors contributing to outbreaks of food poisoning in England and Wales 1970–79. *J. Hygiene*, 89, 491
6. Department of Education and Science (1978) Circular 11/78. *Medical fitness of teachers and entrants to teacher training*. (London: HMSO)
7. Dann, T. C. (1969). Routine skin preparation before injection; an unnecessary procedure. *Lancet*, 2, 96
8. Smith, R. E. (1971). Great school doctors and the evolution of adolescent medicine. *Practitioner*, 206, 183

9. Cmnd 6684 (1976). *Fit for the Future,* Vol. 1. The Report of the Committee on Child Health Services, p.150. (London: HMSO)
10. Illingworth, R. S. (1982). *Basic Developmental Screening: 0–5 years.* 3rd Edn. (Oxford: Blackwell Scientific Publications)
11. Betts, P. (1981). Growth failure. *Br. Med. J.,* 283, 1611
12. Briscoe, J. H. D. (1982). Evaluation of the routine medical examination of 13-year-old 'public school' pupils. *Publ. Hlth. Lond.,* 96, 231

CHAPTER 3

IMMUNIZATION

Introduction

Immunization plays an important part in the prevention of infectious diseases in children. Those concerned with their health have a responsibility in the matter which embraces health education, administration, treatment and communication with the pupils and their parents. They should be satisfied with nothing less than complete efficiency in compiling immunization histories and schedules which ensure that the appropriate procedures are carried out when due. There is an additional responsibility towards the numerous schoolchildren who travel abroad or live overseas.

Many areas have computerized immunization schedules which notify parents when their children's immunizations are due. Records of immunization status may therefore be held centrally, and in a day school the responsibility will be shared with the general practitioner and school medical service (which may, in particular, be involved with BCG and rubella immunization). In most boarding schools the school doctor has an undivided responsibility. A full record of immunizations should be kept and the parents informed of the child's protective state, and parents should be instructed to advise the school doctor of any immunization given in the holidays.

The Medical Defence Union advises that a consent, obtained in writing from the parents on the child's first admission to the school, gives the school doctor, without further reference to the parents, authority to carry out any necessary routine immunizations during the time the child remains in the care of the school doctor. A specimen consent form is given in Appendix B, p. 193. For immunizations not specifically recommended by the Joint Committee on Vaccination and Immunization (JCVI)[1] – for example, influenza and mumps – individual consent is advisable.

A personal record is essential for each child and a copy should be in his or her own possession; this is particularly important in respect of tetanus toxoid. The immunization history should be passed on in the NHS medical envelope when the child leaves the school, and a copy retained as a permanent record. Immunization records must also be available to the teaching staff (see p. 7).

Vaccine-induced immunity

Immunity can be induced against an increasing variety of bacterial and viral agents or their products, and may be passive or active.

Passive immunity results from injecting antiserum containing specific antibodies; this may be obtained from an animal or another human being. It is short-lived, lasting only until the antiserum has been eliminated from the body.

Active immunity provides protection for months or years. It can be induced by the administration of vaccines containing an attenuated living organism of the disease concerned, as in oral poliomyelitis and measles vaccines, or by giving one in which the

Table 1   Vaccines for active immunization (after Welsby[2])

Live vaccines	Measles
	Mumps
	Poliomyelitis (Sabin type)
	Rubella
	Tuberculosis (BCG)
	Yellow Fever
Vaccines prepared from inactivated bacterial cells or their components	Anthrax
	Cholera
	Meningococcal meningitis
	Plague
	Pneumococcal infections
	Typhoid
	Typhus
	Whooping cough
Vaccines prepared from inactivated viral cells or their components	Hepatitis B
	Influenza
	Poliomyelitis (Salk type)
	Rabies
Toxoid preparations	Diphtheria
	Tetanus

organism has been inactivated during manufacture, as in whooping cough and typhoid vaccine. Active immunization against tetanus and diphtheria is produced by toxoids which are devoid of organisms but contain the bacterial toxins rendered harmless by treatment with formaldehyde. All these vaccines, apart from BCG (the bacillus of Calmette and Guérin, which is an attenuated growth of a bovine strain of tubercle bacillus) produce protection by stimulating the production of specific antibodies. Protection afforded by BCG is thought to depend on a cell-mediated immunity mechanism. An important additional effect of oral poliomyelitis vaccine is the development of local immunity in the intestine. Vaccines currently available for passive and active immunization are listed in Tables 1 and 2.

The first dose of an inactivated vaccine or toxoid usually produces only a small, slow antibody response – the 'primary response'. When, after a suitable interval, a second dose is given, the response is quicker and to a higher level – the 'secondary response'. Following a course of active immunization the antibody level may remain high for months or years, but even after this falls off the antibody-producing system remains sensitized, so that a further dose of vaccine will elicit another secondary response.

It is for the individual doctor to decide on the type, dosage and exact timing of the vaccines used, although there is general agreement on the most important aspects. These include the desirability of a basic course of immunization with diphtheria, tetanus, whooping cough, poliomyelitis and measles vaccine during the early years of life, with reinforcing doses of diphtheria, tetanus and

Table 2   Vaccines for passive immunization

Human normal immunoglobulin	Hepatitis A
	Measles
	Rubella
Human specific immunoglobulin	Hepatitis B
	Mumps
	Rabies
	Tetanus
	Varicella/Zoster
Antitoxins	Botulism
	Diphtheria
	Gas gangrene
	Tetanus

Table 3   Schedule of immunization procedures

Age	Vaccines	Interval	Notes
3 months	Diphtheria, tetanus and pertussis triple antigen and oral poliomyelitis vaccine (1st dose)		The first dose is best given at 3 months but may be given at any time during the first year of life. If pertussis vaccine is contraindicated or refused by the parents diphtheria/tetanus vaccine should be given
4½–5 months	Diphtheria, tetanus and pertussis triple antigen and oral poliomyelitis vaccine (2nd dose)	Preferably after 6–8 weeks	
8½–11 months	Diphtheria, tetanus and pertussis triple antigen and oral poliomyelitis vaccine (3rd dose)	Preferably after 4–6 months	
15 months	Measles vaccine	Not less than 3 weeks after another live vaccine	Should be offered to all susceptible children from the second year of life to puberty
At school entry	Diphtheria/tetanus vaccine (4th dose) Oral poliomyelitis vaccine (4th dose)	Preferably at least 3 years after completing primary course	
Between 10 and 13 years	Rubella vaccine – girls only		All girls of this age should be offered rubella vaccine, irrespective of a history of rubella unless known to be sero-positive
Between 10 and 13 years of age	BCG vaccine	Not less than 3 weeks between BCG and rubella vaccination	For tuberculin-negative children and tuberculin-negative contacts at any age
Between 15 and 19 years of age	Tetanus and oral poliomyelitis vaccine (reinforcing dose)	Preferably 10 years after school entry dose	Tetanus vaccine should not be given if a previous dose has been given within the past 5 years

poliomyelitis vaccines at school entry. A further reinforcing dose of tetanus toxoid and poliomyelitis vaccine at 15–19 years of age, or when leaving school, is also advised. BCG is offered to all tuberculin negative pupils between the ages of 10 and 13 inclusive, and rubella to all girls in the same age group.

Contraindications to immunization must always be borne in mind. No vaccine should be given during an acute febrile illness. Live vaccines should not normally be given in pregnancy or to immunocompromised patients, those on steroids, or those receiving radiotherapy. An interval of three weeks should be allowed between the administration of two live vaccines. Specific contraindications are dealt with below in relation to each vaccine.

Routine immunization

The schedule recommended by the JCVI for the routine immunization of children is given in Table 3.

Diphtheria

Reliable immunity is produced by the standard primary course and 5-year-old reinforcing dose of diphtheria formol toxoid, usually given in triple antigen and diphtheria/tetanus vaccine. Formol toxoid should not be given over the age of 10 years without a preliminary Schick test, as it may cause unpleasant local reactions. An adsorbed vaccine for this age group is now available and can safely be given without Schick testing.

Tetanus

Tetanus toxoid provides very long-lasting immunity, and the schedule of a primary course in infancy followed by reinforcing doses at 5 years and 15 years gives protection well into middle life. Difficulties often arise in deciding whether to give a reinforcing dose following an injury. Hypersensitivity reactions occur when unnecessarily frequent doses of tetanus toxoid are given, sometimes because the immunization history is not known. It is generally accepted that a reinforcing dose should not be given less than 5 years after a previous dose; this illustrates the importance of personal immunization records and accessible school immunization records.

When an injury occurs to someone who has not been immunized with tetanus toxoid, specific human antitetanus immunoglobulin (Humotet) should be given if the wound has not been treated within 6 hours of injury and is potentially heavily contaminated with tetanus spores: puncture wounds and those with much devitalized tissue are particularly at risk. In such cases 250 units of immuno-globulin should be given with the first dose of a course of tetanus toxoid.

Whooping cough

Controversy continues over whether or not there is a syndrome leading to brain damage following whooping cough vaccine affect-ing between 1 in 17 000 and 1 in 52 000 vaccinated children[3]. In the context of school health, the question of pertussis vaccination only arises in those children who have not been given it in infancy. Following the epidemic of whooping cough consequent on low vaccine uptake rates, many parents seek advice about having a primary course when the children are older. The main advantage of this is the protection of infant siblings to whom the unimmunized child may transmit whooping cough. It is now recommended that vaccine can be given to children up to their 6th birthday, as a 3-dose course of monovalent pertussis vaccine (plain or adsorbed) at monthly intervals.

The JCVI advises[1] that whooping cough vaccination should not be carried out in children who have a history of any severe local or general reaction (including a neurological reaction) to a preceding dose, or in children with a history of cerebral irritation or damage in the neonatal period, or those who have suffered from convulsions. There are other groups of children in whom whooping cough vacci-nation is not absolutely contraindicated but who require special consideration as to its advisability. These are children whose par-ents or siblings have a history of idiopathic epilepsy, children with developmental delay thought to be due to a neurological defect, and children with neurological disease. As the risks of vaccination may be higher than normal in these children, the balance of risks of whooping cough and vaccine should be carefully weighed.

Poliomyelitis

Live attenuated (Sabin type) oral vaccine is used almost exclusively in the United Kingdom, and contains virus types 1, 2 and 3. There is a very small theoretical risk of the virus acquiring virulence by passage through the gut, and for this reason it is advised that unimmunized parents should receive vaccine at the same time as their children. Inactivated (Salk type) vaccine is available from the DHSS for pregnant women and others for whom live vaccine is contraindicated.

Measles

Measles vaccine is normally given in the second year of life, as natural immunity may interfere with its efficacy before this. The protection afforded appears to be lifelong, except in those in whom vaccine fails to produce antibodies. These amount to about 5%, but when measles occurs in this group it is milder than in the unvaccinated to a statistically significant degree[4]. The policy of vaccination has ended the two-year cycle of epidemics which used to occur, so that an increasing number of unvaccinated children reach secondary school age unprotected. It is well worth vaccinating any schoolchildren up to the age of 15 who are found to be without measles antibody; if the antibody status is unknown those who have not been vaccinated or had an attack of measles should be offered vaccination. Mild reactions with malaise, fever and a rash may occur 5–10 days after vaccination. Specific contraindications are children with untreated active tuberculosis, and those hypersensitive to polymyxin or neomycin. Children with a history of convulsions or whose mother, father or siblings have a history of idiopathic epilepsy should be given specially diluted human normal immunoglobulin simultaneously.

Measles vaccine can also be given to susceptible contacts to control an outbreak, as soon as possible after the diagnosis of the index case.

Rubella

The policy in the United Kingdom, which differs radically from that in the USA, is to allow rubella outbreaks to continue among males and prepubertal girls, giving a good chance of natural immunity to be acquired, and to ensure the safety of girls by rubella vaccination between their 10th and 14th birthdays. There is now good evidence that this protects throughout reproductive life. As studies have shown very poor correlation between a history of rubella and the presence of antibody, rubella vaccine is recommended for all girls irrespective of their supposed history. Mild reactions to vaccine are common, especially in adults: they consist of fever, rash, lymphadenopathy, arthralgia and sometimes transient polyarthritis. Where the rubella antibody level is known, as in schools participating in research programmes such as the Study of Influenza in Residential Schools, vaccine need not be given to those found to have naturally-acquired antibody.

The prevention of congenital rubella depends upon a high uptake of rubella vaccine, and health authorities and school doctors have an obligation to do everything in their power to achieve a response rate as near 100% as possible. A survey[5] in the early years of rubella vaccination showed poor rates in girls educated in independent schools. It is doubtful whether the same results would be found today, but the challenge to doctors of independent schools must not be ignored.

Vaccination is not offered routinely to women of child-bearing age because there is a theoretical possibility that harm to the fetus could follow if pregnancy occurred within the following 12 weeks. Teachers, nurses and staff in schools may be at risk of contracting rubella, and it is therefore advisable that all women in these groups should have their antibody status determined; if found to be seronegative they should be offered vaccination, provided they are fully aware of the need to avoid pregnancy for the next 3 months.

BCG

There is still sufficient pulmonary tuberculosis in the country for BCG vaccination of schoolchildren to remain official policy in the United Kingdom. It is given routinely to 10–13 year old children who are tuberculin negative. As the risk is greatest among immigrant families, the Joint Tuberculosis Committee of the British Tuberculosis Association recommends that children born in the United Kingdom of immigrant parents should be given BCG at birth. Children arriving in the country from Asia and Africa should be tuberculin tested and negative reactors should be given BCG vaccination.

There are a number of tuberculin tests in current use, the Mantoux, Heaf, Tine and Imotest, all of which use a preparation of tuberculo-protein, usually in the form of purified protein derivate (PPD) introduced into the skin. A positive response indicates previous exposure to mycobacteria or active mycobacterial infection. Positive reactors should not be given BCG vaccine but must be followed up by means of chest X-ray. Even if the chest X-ray is normal, there is a case for giving chemotherapy to those with strongly positive reactions, especially children from overseas. Those with a negative response (including a Grade 1 Heaf test) should be vaccinated with 0.1 ml BCG vaccine. It is important that this should be given intradermally, as subcutaneous injection can lead to abscess formation. BCG vaccination is contraindicated in the presence of local sepsis. No further immunization should be given in the same arm for at least 3 months because of the risk of regional lymphadenitis. Some virus infections, such as measles, rubella and chickenpox, can suppress the tuberculin test for 4–6 weeks, so tuberculin testing should not be carried out in the 6 weeks after rubella or measles vaccination, and BCG should not be given for 3 weeks after these vaccinations. As rubella and BCG vaccination are carried out at about the same age, school programmes should be drawn up with these considerations in mind.

Mumps

A live attenuated mumps vaccine is available, but is little used in the United Kingdom compared with the USA. There is a case for giving it to boys who are found to be antibody-negative in secondary school, as the disease can be most unpleasant in postpubertal males, with orchitis a not uncommon complication. Antibody studies give strong reason to believe that protection will be lifelong. The only specific contraindication is hypersensitivity to neomycin.

Influenza

Killed influenza vaccines are prepared in chick embryos from whole or split viruses. Their usefulness is limited by the constant changes of the surface antigens of influenza A virus and the difficulties of manufacturing vaccine fast enough to keep up with these changes. After the reappearance of the H_1N_1 virus in December 1977, for example, the first available vaccine arrived too late to prevent massive outbreaks in a totally susceptible school population. When the appropriate vaccine can be given, protection rates varying from 40 to 70% have been demonstrated. In these circumstances, the impact of influenza epidemics in boarding schools can be reduced and this was the basis for the enthusiasm with which annual influenza vaccination was embraced in the 1960s[6]. This enthusiasm has now been tempered by increasing knowledge of the limitations of vaccination. In any one year, a large proportion of the school population may already have acquired immunity from previous infection, and therefore derive no benefit from vaccination; furthermore, the vaccine may not contain the strain which subsequently causes outbreaks, or the expected epidemic may never come, as with the 'swine influenza' alert in 1976. One study[7] has suggested that, in the case of H_3N_2 influenza, vaccination with the appropriate strain did no more than postpone the attack until further antigenic drift had occurred. Revaccination produces very little rise in antibody level, so it is unlikely that any further protection is obtained by vaccinating the same people repeatedly.

Opinions on the use of influenza vaccine in schools therefore remain divided, and the matter is one in which schools are co-operating in continuing research. An effective vaccine would certainly be a boon, and the future may lie in the development of live vaccines.

The World Health Organization makes recommendations each year on which strains are to be included in influenza vaccines, and these currently contain representatives of the three main subtypes in circulation, $A(H_1N_1)$, $A(H_3N_2)$ and B. They are mainly recommended for those at high risk from chronic pulmonary, cardiovascular and renal disease and diabetes. The JCVI does not recommend vaccination for the attempted control of the general spread of influenza. Influenza vaccine is contraindicated in those sensitive to egg protein and feathers.

Hepatitis B

Hepatitis B vaccine, prepared from the plasma of human carriers, is in short supply and expensive. The JCVI at present recommends that its use should be restricted to health care personnel who are likely to be in contact with high risk carriers, and to certain patients and family contacts, including haemophiliacs and patients on first entry to institutions for the mentally handicapped where there is known to be a high incidence of hepatitis B. There is no need to give the vaccine to individuals known to be hepatitis B surface antigen (or antibody) positive.

Smallpox

The world was declared free of smallpox in December 1979, and this declaration was ratified by the World Health Assembly in 1980.

Smallpox vaccine carries a small but definite risk, and there is therefore no longer any medical justification for using it. The only exceptions are investigators and staff working on smallpox virus and those who have agreed to man any hospital which will be designated to deal with patients strongly suspected of having smallpox.

Pneumococcal pneumonia

A polyvalent vaccine is available for use in those whose risk of contracting pneumococcal pneumonia is unusually high, such as patients who have had a splenectomy. The present vaccine contains the 14 most prevalent types of pneumococcus. Protection probably lasts about 5 years.

Prophylaxis for overseas travel

The school doctor's advice on overseas travel may be required in the planning of overseas expeditions and in the supervision of boarding school pupils whose parents live or work overseas. This section is concerned with the immunization implications of travel and the imperative need for malaria prophylaxis, but it is most important that intending travellers overseas should be aware that no prophylactic measures provide absolute protection. In the countries where poliomyelitis, typhoid, cholera or any other gastrointestinal illnesses are common, strict attention to personal hygiene is important. Salads and uncooked vegetables should be avoided, fruit should be peeled at the time of eating and no untreated water should be used for drinking or cleaning teeth. For a fuller account of the health implications of overseas travel the reader is referred to the Ross Institute's publication *Preservation of Personal Health in Warm Climates*[8]. No specific immunizations are required for travel to North America. Northern Europe or Australasia. The DHSS provides detailed information on the recommendations for other countries in Leaflet SA35, *Notice to travellers*[9].

International certificates

The only international vaccination certificate still officially in force is for yellow fever. Many countries still demand cholera certificates, however, despite the fact that the World Health Organization discontinued them in 1973. The old international certificate forms are still available, and should be used for those countries which require them.

Poliomyelitis

Of all the vaccines required for travel outside Europe, poliomyelitis is the most often forgotten, and may well be the most important, as the disease is still prevalent in many warm countries. If it has not been given within the previous 5 years a reinforcing dose should be given.

Tetanus

Tetanus is no more or less a risk to travellers than to others, but in planning an immunization programme for a traveller, the opportunity should not be lost to confirm that tetanus immunization is up to date: a reinforcing dose within the past 10 years is sufficient for those who have had a primary course.

Measles

As with tetanus, it is a wise precaution to check the immune status of a child before travelling, particularly to those countries where measles is particularly virulent.

Typhoid

Typhoid prophylaxis is given in the form of monovalent typhoid vaccine prepared from a killed suspension of *Salmonella typhi* organisms. TAB vaccine, containing *Salmonella paratyphi* A and B organisms in addition, is no longer used, as the paratyphoid vaccine is of dubious value and the combined vaccine is more likely to give rise to local reactions. Two doses of 0.5 ml should be given by deep subcutaneous or intramuscular injection, at an interval of 4–6 weeks, and where necessary reinforcing doses every 3 years will maintain antibody levels. For children under 10, 0.25 ml should be given. Second and subsequent doses can be given intradermally in a dose of 0.1 ml: protection appears to be comparable with other routes, and the likelihood of local reaction is diminished.

Attempts are being made to produce a live vaccine which should be more effective than the killed vaccine.

Cholera

Unfortunately, the main indication for giving cholera vaccine is to meet the requirements of those countries demanding so-called international vaccination certificates, which are valid for only 6 months. The vaccine is of limited potency, and the main protection against cholera in people visiting areas where it is endemic is attention to the hygiene of the food and water they consume. The vaccine is given subcutaneously or intramuscularly in a dose of 0.5 ml (0.3 ml for children aged 6–10 years, 0.1 ml for those aged 1–5 years), or intradermally in a dose of 0.1 ml. The second dose of 1 ml (0.5 ml for children aged 6–10 years, 0.3 ml aged 1–5 years) or 0.2 ml intradermally (0.1 ml for children) can be given within a week to satisfy certificate requirements, but is better given after 4 weeks. The duration of immunity is short-lived, and for repeated travel to countries requiring vaccination certificates reinforcing doses must be given every 6 months.

Yellow fever

Yellow fever vaccine is a live attenuated vaccine which is given only in special centres. It is required for travel to most areas of Africa and Central South America between the latitudes of 15°N and 15°S. The international certificate is valid for 10 years. Details of yellow fever vaccination centres in the United Kingdom are given in the DHSS *Notice to travellers*[9].

Hepatitis A

Passive protection against infectious hepatitis with human gamma globulin is only advised where the degree of exposure to infection is likely to be high, or when the patient, if infected, may be less resistant on account of pre-existing disease. The recommended dose is 0.02–0.04 ml/kg bodyweight by deep intramuscular injection, giving protection for about 2 months. If continuous protection is needed up to 6 months in adults, a dose four times as large is recommended, leading to bulky, painful intramuscular injections.

Rabies

A human diploid cell rabies vaccine is available for the protection of those at high risk, such as veterinary surgeons and workers in quarantine kennels. It is not generally recommended for preexposure immunization of travellers, partly on account of its high cost. Nevertheless, for those who have to spend some time in areas of high risk, a case can be argued for prophylactic immunization[10]. It must be paid for by the patient, who may feel the cost is justified by the peace of mind it brings.

Typhus

An inactivated vaccine gives protection for those likely to be living in close personal contact with the indigenous population of an area where typhus is endemic. It is available from the DHSS for named patients only.

Plague

A killed vaccine is available for laboratory workers and those spending some time in rural areas with enzootic or epidemic plague. Among schoolchildren this must be a rare circumstance. The epidemiology of plague, which is covered by WHO Health Regulations, was reviewed in 1983 by the Communicable Disease Surveillance Centre[11].

The 'late' patient

School doctors are sometimes requested to immunize children going abroad at short notice, when it is too late for the correct intervals to be allowed to elapse. No hard and fast rules can be laid down. Single doses of typhoid or cholera vaccine are effective if the subject has previously had the two doses course, and even if the child has not been previously immunized a single dose is better than none. There is no objection to double inoculations on the same day in cases of urgency.

Malaria prophylaxis

Malaria prophylaxis has assumed increasing importance, with the number of cases diagnosed in the United Kingdom having risen to 2000 annually in the late 1970s and drug resistance spreading to ever wider areas. The disease is present in many parts of Africa, Central and South America, Asia and Oceania. Details are readily available in the DHSS *Notice to travellers*[9] and medical periodicals. In many areas falciparum malaria is resistant to chloroquine, so that drug regimes are under constant review. In cases of doubt the DHSS and the Institute of Tropical Medicine will advise by telephone on the choice of prophylactics for given areas.

Prophylactic drugs should be started a week before departure, to allow time to change drugs in case of a reaction, and to establish the habit of taking antimalarials, and should be continued for at least a month after leaving the malarious area.

In chloroquine-sensitive areas, the drug of choice is either proguanil 200 mg daily or chloroquine 300 mg base weekly. In areas where chloroquine-resistant falciparum malaria is present, one tablet of Fansidar (pyrimethamine 25 mg + sulfadoxine 500 mg) or Maloprim (pyrimethamine 12.5 mg + dapsone 100 mg) should be taken once a week. Both of these drugs are less effective against the benign forms of malaria, so that when *Plasmodium vivax* and chloroquine-resistant *Plasmodium falciparum* coexist, chloroquine 300 mg base should be added to the weekly dose. The doses given are for 12-year-olds and over. Three-quarters of the adult dose is recommended for those between 20 and 40 kg, half the adult dose for those between 5 and 20 kg, and a quarter of the adult dose for infants under 5 kg.

There are now some areas where Fansidar-resistance has been reported, so authoritative local advice or DHSS advice should be taken. Fansidar is contraindicated in sulphonamide sensitivity.

The centres from which further advice can be obtained are as follows:

DHSS, London	01-407 5522, ext. 6711/6749
Ross Institute of Tropical Hygiene, London	01-636 8636
School of Tropical Medicine, Liverpool	051-708 9393
East Birmingham Hospital	021-772 4311
Ruchill Hospital, Glasgow	041-946 7120

References

1. Joint Committee on Vaccination and Immunization (1982). *Immunization Against Infectious Disease*. (London: DHSS)
2. Welsby, P.D. (1981). *Infectious Diseases*. (Lancaster: MTP Press)
3. Pollock, T.M. and Morris, J. (1983). A 7-year survey of disorders attributed to vaccination in North West Thames Region. *Lancet*, 1, 753
4. Measles Sub-Committee of the Committee on Development of Vaccines and Immunisation Procedures (1977). Clinical trial of live measles vaccine given alone and live vaccine preceded by killed vaccine. *Lancet*, 2, 571

5. Peckham, C.S., Marshall, S.C. and Dudgeon, J.A. (1977). Rubella vaccination of schoolgirls: factors affecting vaccine uptake. *Br. Med. J.*, 1, 760
6. Turtle, P. de B. (1968). Vaccines in the management of influenza epidemics in schools. *Practitioner*, 200, 254
7. Hoskins, T. W., Davies, J. R., Smith, A. J., Miller, C. L. and Allchin, A. (1979). Assessment of inactivated influenza A vaccine after three outbreaks of influenza A at Christ's Hospital. *Lancet*, 1, 33
8. Ross Institute of Tropical Hygiene (1980). *Preservation of Personal Health in Warm Climates*. 8th Edn. (London: Ross Institute of Tropical Hygiene)
9. Department of Health and Social Security (1984). *Protect your Health Abroad. Notice to Travellers*. Leaflet SA35. (London: DHSS)
10. Anonymous (1983). Rabies. *Lancet*, 1, 967
11. PHLS Communicable Disease Surveillance Centre (1983). Plague. *Commun. Dis. Rep.* 83/17, 3

CHAPTER 4

CHILDHOOD AND ADOLESCENCE

The physical development of prepubertal children

It is not the intention of this Handbook to attempt to summarize the large literature on developmental paediatrics, but as some children begin to attend nursery school in the third year of life, it is appropriate to give some points of reference. All concerned with the healthy development of the schoolchild are permanently indebted to the work of Mary Sheridan. Appendix E, p. 200, reproduces the part of her chart which deals with average attainments in the nursery school age-group. It should not be applied uncritically, and those using it are urged to consult the brief but cogent introduction to *The Developmental Progress of Infants and Young Children*[1]. The author emphasizes that the chart is not intended to produce a quotient of any sort, and the words 'pass' and 'fail' are inappropriate.

The other British authority whose name is almost synonymous with the study of growth in childhood and adolescence is J. M. Tanner, whose *Education and Physical Growth*[2] summarizes the implications of his work for 'teachers and lecturers in colleges, institutes and university departments of education, and all whose professional and personal interests make them concerned with our educational system'. Much of what follows draws inevitably on his writings and charts, which are reproduced in most textbooks of paediatrics.

From the age of 5 years until the beginning of the adolescent growth spurt, the growth rate of children is fairly constant (Figure 1).

The physical changes of puberty

The adolescent growth spurt in the average girl begins at about $10\frac{1}{2}$ years and reaches its maximum at 12 years, with menarche occurring at $12\frac{1}{2}$ years. The whole process of puberty takes about 3 years. In the average boy it takes place 18 months to 2 years later, and lasts

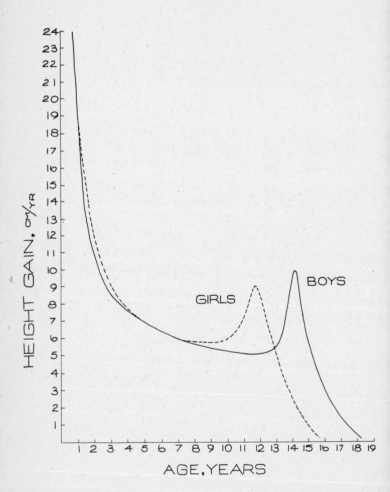

Figure 1   Average height velocity curves for boys and girls (from Tanner *et al.* (1966). *Arch. Dis. Child.* **)**

slightly longer. These average figures conceal a striking individual variation, with the result that any sizeable group of 12-year-old girls or 14-year-old boys will include prepubertal and almost fully mature individuals. This is illustrated in Figure 2. As mental capacity develops roughly in parallel with physical size, the difference between the sexes and the range of individual variation have important implications for teachers as well as games instructors.

Most measurements of the body increase at much the same rate as body height, with some exceptions illustrated in Figure 3. The brain and skull develop earlier than other parts of the body, while lymphatic tissue diminishes in size after puberty. The eyeball keeps pace with brain development, but a small adolescent spurt in the axial length of the eye probably accounts for the fact that myopia so

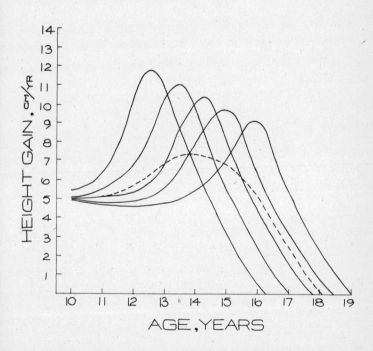

Figure 2   Height velocity curves of five boys in the Harpenden Growth Study. The dotted line shows the 'average' velocity obtained by plotting the mean values, thus smoothing out the true adolescent growth spurt (from Tanner *et al.* (1966). *Arch. Dis. Child.*)

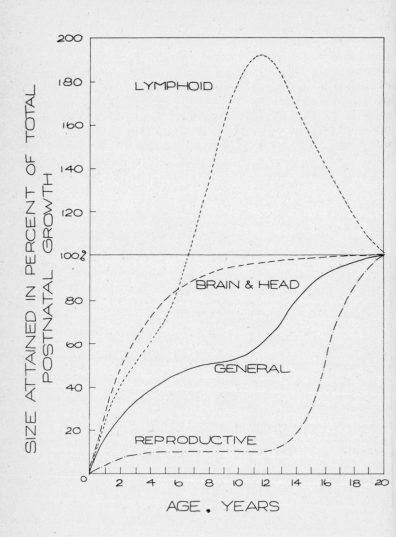

Figure 3   Growth curves of different parts of the body (from Tanner (1962). *Growth at Adolescence*)

often develops at the time of puberty. The facial measurements change rapidly in adolescence and facial expression changes markedly, especially in boys.

The hands and feet are the next after the skull to reach adult size. Leg length then begins to increase rapidly, and this is the stage at which coltish adolescents are at their most clumsy. However, most of the height spurt is due to subsequent trunk growth. Girls have a particularly large spurt in hip width, while boys increase most in shoulder breadth. Muscle, including heart muscle, grows rapidly in mass and strength, more so in boys than girls, and there is a considerable increase in athletic ability. Boys tend to lose fat, but girls do not.

The increased secretion of gonadotrophins from the pituitary

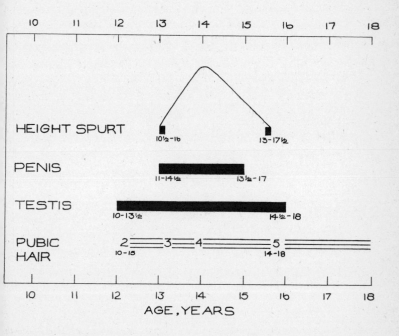

Figure 4 Diagram of sequence of events at adolescence in boys, showing the average and the range of ages at which each stage is reached (from Tanner (1962). *Growth at Adolescence*)

leads in turn to the development of the sex organs in a sequence illustrated in Figures 4 and 5. Tanner has devised a simple five-point scale of development of genitalia, pubic hair and breast which is useful in recording the stage of development reached at a given time. This is given in Appendix E (p. 204) together with Tanner's charts for the heights and weights of boys and girls.

Menstruation

It will be seen from Figure 5 that menarche generally follows the onset of breast development by about 2 years. The enlightened attitude to menstruation which is now usual amongst girls and in schools was first widely disseminated 60 years ago by Dr A.

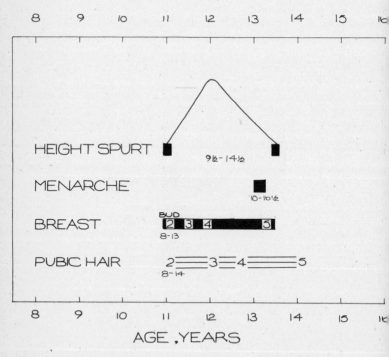

Figure 5   **Diagram of sequence of events at adolescence in girls, showing the average and the range of ages at which each stage is reached (from Tanner (1962).** *Growth at Adolescence*)

Sanderson Clow, Medical Officer to Cheltenham Ladies' College[3]. It is still undermined occasionally by mothers and even housemistresses who cling to the old idea of unwellness and the need for extra care. School doctors can do much to encourage a more realistic approach. If women are to take their full place in life, whether in work or sport, the variation of the menstrual cycle cannot be allowed to interfere with their lives. On the other hand, spasmodic dysmenorrhoea can be very disabling, and its management is discussed in Chapter 5 (p. 85).

Internal protection for the menstrual flow is now widely used and helps towards the maintenance of normal activity. The use of tampons by girls should no longer be discouraged and most cope remarkably well. If, however, a girl in her late teens is worried or distressed by being unable to insert them expert help should be sought. Vaginismus or anatomical abnormality may be the cause and can usually be overcome. (It is worth mentioning here that any woman who has failed to insert tampons should seek advice and the difficulty be corrected before marriage; otherwise non-consummation may wreck the union.) A forgotten tampon produces a very offensive vaginal discharge, but removal is all that is required.

A recent problem has arisen in connection with tampons in that a few cases of toxic shock syndrome associated with vaginal infection have been reported, the majority from the USA. Most but not all of these have coincided with menstruation and most of the patients have been wearing tampons at the time. As internal protection is now used by the vast majority of women the possible implications of these cases require statistical evaluation. The considered opinion in this country is that 'there is no justification at present for any suggestion that women should avoid using tampons since the risk of developing toxic shock syndrome is extremely small'[4].

The emotional changes of adolescence

The concept of adolescence as a period of transition from childhood to adulthood goes back to Aristotle, but the idea that it is usually a period of storm and stress dates only from the beginning of the present century. The secular trend towards earlier puberty – the average age at menarche has fallen 3 years in the past century – combined with the ever-increasing length of the period of schooling, may have some bearing on changing attitudes towards adolescence, which some see as largely culturally determined.

The psychoanalytic school helped to mould a view of adolescence which can be summarized in a passage by Anna Freud:[5]

'I take it that it is normal for an adolescent to behave for a considerable length of time in an inconsistent and unpredictable manner; to fight his impulses and to accept them; to ward them off successfully and to be overrun by them; to love his parents and to hate them; to revolt against them and be dependent on them; to be deeply ashamed to acknowledge his mother before others and, unexpectedly, to desire heart-to-heart talks with her; to thrive on imitation or identification with others while searching unceasingly for his own identity; to be more idealistic, artistic, generous and unselfish than he will ever be again, but also the opposite; self-centred, egoistic, calculating. Such fluctuations between opposites would be deemed highly abnormal at any other time of life. At this time they may signify no more than that an adult structure of personality takes a long time to emerge'.

The author went so far as to suggest that it was abnormal and possibly dangerous when an adolescent 'showed no outer evidence of inner unrest'. Erikson[6,7] developed the idea of the identity crisis alluded to in the above passage. Miller[8] concisely defined identity as 'a conscious sense of individual uniqueness', the development of which can be preceded by a period of extreme psychic turbulence, often lasting about 6 months.

All of these concepts, developed by therapists whose main experience of adolescents was of those referred to them in varying states of psychic turbulence, are unmistakably descriptive of the emotional processes of some adolescents. Rutter set out, in a careful study in the Isle of Wight, to determine to what extent they are representative of normal adolescent development. A random sample of 10% of all 14 and 15-year-old boys and girls living in the Isle of Wight in 1968 and 1969 were interviewed in depth, and their parents were interviewed separately. The results were presented in the 1979 Rock Carling lecture and published by the Nuffield Provincial Hospitals Trust[9]. This monograph should be consulted for the detailed data, but the striking conclusion was 'Normal adolescence is *not* characterized by storm, stress and disturbance. Most young people go through their teenage years without significant emotional or behavioural problems'. The generation gap, for instance, was found to be less marked between the adolescents studied and their parents than between the parents and *their* parents. Rutter found, nevertheless, that more than a fifth of the adolescents reported that they felt miserable and depressed, and that teachers and parents were often unaware of the young people's inner turmoil, perhaps because of their preference for confiding in their own age-group.

Adults involved with those negotiating the period of adolescence, therefore, will find the classical descriptions of its conflicts enlightening for the small minority, but should acknowledge with relief Rutter's discovery that most adolescents negotiate this exciting period of transition without much difficulty. The less fortunate minority are the ones to whom the caring professions necessarily devote much time, and to whom most space in books of this kind has to be devoted.

In the development of emotional attachments in adolescence, Tereschenko, quoted by Hadfield [10], usefully described four phases which are commonly encountered. First, in early adolescence there is attachment to a group of the same sex, leading to the tendency for boys to go about in gangs and girls to congregate with a group of friends. Members of male gangs measure their masculinity against each other in terms of physical strength, athletic prowess and genital endowment. The second phase is attachment to an individual of the same sex, who may be of the same age or a considerably older person who may be the object of hero worship or a 'crush'. The third phase is attachment to a group of the opposite sex, and the fourth is attachment to an individual of the opposite sex, an attachment which is frequently idealistic and platonic at first. At that stage, the individual is ready to strive towards the maturity in which genital love can flourish. Erikson [7] describes the ultimate goal of love as the Utopia of genitality, a Utopia which not everyone may wish to achieve. It should include, he says,

'(1)   mutuality of orgasm,
 (2)   with a loved partner,
 (3)   of the other sex,
 (4)   with whom one is able and willing to share a mutual trust,
 (5)   and with whom one is able and willing to regulate the cycles of
           (a)   work
           (b)   procreation
           (c)   recreation,
 (6)   so as to secure to the offspring, too, all stages of a satisfactory development'.

Some problems of adolescents at school

Anorexia nervosa

Anorexia nervosa is most commonly encountered among boarding school girls from socioeconomic classes I and II. Its increased incidence in recent years may be related to the fashion for dieting, but as Dally and Gomez[11] point out, 'While the pursuit of thinness is a sociocultural phenomenon that forms the backcloth to anorexia nervosa, the reasons for its development vary from one patient to another'. There is convincing evidence that it can be seen as a phobia of body shape[12]. It has been shown that within fairly small limits menstruation ceases when the weight falls below 47 kg, and follicular stimulating and luteinizing hormones cease to circulate below 43 kg, with a consequent loss of sexual feelings. The development of anorexia nervosa can thus be a means of avoiding the stresses of sexual maturation.

There are varieties of anorexia nervosa, including bingeing and bulimia and purging, and the much rarer male condition, but the classical picture is of the girl who loses weight excessively and ceases to menstruate. She is generally full of energy, obsessed with food of which she does not herself partake, compliant, hardworking, conscientious and meticulous. She will deny that there is any problem, but family anxiety may be considerable.

Undoubtedly many minor cases occur and recover spontaneously. Such girls can be helped by monitoring their weight and ensuring that regular meals are taken. In the more severe cases, organic causes should be excluded, but these are very seldom found. A target weight, based on the mean matched population weight, should be set and must not be negotiable. Lacy[13] recommends a normal school diet supplemented by two rounds of cheese sandwiches daily as a good source of extra calories. Psychotherapy may be helpful.

In severe cases hospital admission for a long period may be necessary. If vomiting occurs or bodyweight falls by more than 25%, admission is indicated as there is an appreciable mortality, equally distributed between simple inanition and suicide.

Self-poisoning and attempted suicide

In adolescent girls suicide attempts succeed in only about 1%, and some writers therefore prefer to use the term parasuicide for an increasingly common phenomenon which for some girls replaces language as a means of communicating their anger or despair. The incidence of self-poisoning is strongly correlated with the level of prescribing of psychotrophic drugs, so the school doctor can play a part in prevention by extreme caution in using them, particularly as epidemics of self-poisoning sometimes occur in schools. The management of a case of attempted suicide begins with resuscitation and psychiatric assessment in hospital. The opportunity must not be missed for counselling the patient and, where possible, her family. It may be thought unnecessary to state that psychotrophic drugs should not play a part in the subsequent management, yet repeated attempts are too often made with drugs prescribed in the hospital where the first attempt was treated. Overdoses are much less common in boys than girls. Suicide attempts, whether successful or not, may of course occur as a symptom of severe psychiatric disorder, but as the onset of the psychoses generally occurs after school age, this is a rarity in school practice.

School refusal

School refusal is a form of separation anxiety in which a child refuses to go to school and often has a plethora of psychosomatic symptoms such as abdominal pain, headaches, nausea and diarrhoea. The psychopathology usually lies in the mother–child relationship, and the longer absence from school is allowed to continue the more difficult the problem is to resolve. The child needs to be firmly returned to school by the parents with the support and active assistance of the school staff, social worker or psychotherapist. Family psychotherapy is needed to explore and resolve the underlying reasons for the anxiety. In boarding schools, separation anxiety of this kind can result in pathological homesickness and running away. To resolve it, the whole family needs professional help. A contract of weekends at home at increasing intervals is often successful, but in some cases there is no alternative to the child's withdrawal from boarding school, followed by continuing family psychotherapeutic support.

Bullying and mobbing

Aggressive behaviour is an inevitable part of school life, but although it has played a vivid part in novels about the nineteenth century public schools and memoirs of twentieth century literary figures, it has been strangely neglected by educationalists and doctors. Olweus[14] studied bullying in a Swedish school and Orton [15] has drawn attention to the phenomenon of mobbing.

Olweus found that about 5% of a boys' school population could be classed as bullies, and 5% as whipping boys. Contrary to popular belief, the two groups did not overlap but were quite distinct, neither were they significantly below average in academic achievement. The whipping boys tended to be weaker in physical strength and often had over-protective parents, but in other respects (such as physical handicap, obesity and foreign origin) did not differ from a control group. The bullies were characterized by a strong need to dominate, and often had weak relationships with their parents. Although the personality-types are determined before school age, Olweus concludes that there is no place for a tacitly permissive attitude among teachers, who are advised to be authoritative and firm but not punitive.

Mobbing, according to Orton, is a form of non-accidental injury which differs from bullying in being aggression of the group against an individual. Mobbing among boys tends to be physical and among girls psychological. Mobbers are secretive and victims are so cowed that they dare not protest for fear of retribution. Teachers are often unaware and express incredulity when told of what is happening to their pupils. Hemming[16] believes that the antidote to mobbing consists in building up the self-confidence of all adolescents, and criticizes the present educational system which puts a premium on academic achievement and thereby generates failure. Schools should be friendly, purposeful communities with a role of value for every member and physical outlets such as adventure training.

Alcohol, tobacco and drugs

Alcohol

The alcohol consumption of adults in the United Kingdom has doubled since 1950, and it is not surprising that there has been as great a rise in alcohol problems at school.

Ethyl alcohol is a central nervous system depressant, and this results in the well-known effects of disinhibition, impaired skills and impaired judgement. It is also a drug of dependence. Alcoholic drinks have been made since at least 6000 BC by the fermentation of sugars by yeast, which cannot survive once the alcohol concentration reaches 14% by volume. Beers contain between 4 and 8% alcohol, unfortified wines between 8 and 14%, and spirits, which are concentrated by distillation, up to 40%. Liqueurs contain up to 55% alcohol. The absorption of alcohol into the bloodstream takes place most rapidly after taking the more concentrated drinks, and is slowed down when alcohol is accompanied by food because of the slower emptying of the stomach. Very little alcohol is excreted unchanged, although the concentration in the breath correlates well with the blood concentration. 95% of alcohol drunk is distributed to all the tissues of the body, those with the richest blood supply (such as the brain) receiving the highest concentration. Alcohol is metabolized at a rate roughly equivalent to a pint of beer or a double measure of spirits per hour.

Driving skill is affected when the blood alcohol level reaches 30 mg/100 ml, changes in mood and behaviour begin to be apparent at 50 mg/100 ml, driving is seriously affected at 80 mg/100 ml, which is the legal limit in the United Kingdom, and clumsiness and emotional lability develop at 100 mg/100 ml.

At 300 mg/100 ml most individuals are highly intoxicated, leading to stupor. The fatal concentration is 500–800 mg/100 ml, which can be reached by drinking one bottle of spirits. The licensing laws forbid the sale of alcohol to persons under the age of 18 years but they are difficult to enforce.

Drinking among schoolchildren causes concern for two main reasons: the physical and social effects of episodes of drunkenness, and the formation of habits which may lead to long-term damage. Teenagers can be notoriously injudicious in their use of alcohol, and there is a risk of disaster due to alcoholic coma or inhalation of vomit. In a boarding school pupils should, as a matter of policy, be admitted to the sanatorium under professional observation if intoxicated, and this should be seen to be quite separate from any disciplinary action which might be taken, though the doctor may well wish to provide some firm counselling in the cold light of day.

One of the results of the increase in the consumption of alcohol and its decreased cost in real terms is that the habit of heavy drinking is acquired by an increasing number of young people in their teens. This calls for careful health education and the promotion of a responsible attitude towards alcohol, including discussion about total abstinence or moderation in drinking. The Royal College of Psychiatrists[17] suggests that reasonable guidelines for the upper limit of drinking in adults is four pints of beer a day, four doubles of spirits, or one standard-size bottle of wine, but adds that it is unwise to make a habit of drinking even at these levels and that anyone driving a vehicle should not drink at all before driving.

These limits should certainly be revised downwards in advising schoolchildren, who may not realize how readily a regular drinking habit can lead to an increasing daily intake to the point where dependence is acquired.

Tobacco

Now that the many health hazards of tobacco smoking have at last been accepted as established facts, there are signs that the tide is beginning to turn. There are now, for instance, more adult non-smokers than smokers in the United Kingdom. Nevertheless, cigarette smoking remains the most rapidly addictive of all forms of self-gratification, and over a quarter of British schoolchildren are regular smokers by the time they reach the fifth form[18], so that the challenge to those concerned with schoolchildren is as great as ever.

A fairly large body of research[19-21] shows the remarkably early age at which experimentation with smoking begins, the attraction to boys of the image of toughness of the smoker, the influence on them of smoking adults, the negative correlation of smoking behaviour with educational success, and the small impact made on school-children by knowledge of the health risks. It has also shown that the attitude of parents and the school have a considerable effect on whether or not a child becomes a smoker. The greatest contribution that parents and teachers (not to mention doctors and nurses) can therefore make is not to smoke themselves and not to condone the habit in their children and pupils. Next comes education on the effects of smoking on the body, and this is effectively covered in many science courses in schools. Finally comes the general attitude of the community as a caring society which is concerned about smokers' damage to their own health and their lack of consideration towards others. The school doctor should of course play a leading part in promoting this attitude.

Drug abuse

The use and abuse of drugs is as old as mankind, and Edwards[22] reminds us of the many changes of attitude, ranging from approval to abhorrence, in different cultures and different generations towards various types of drug. Experimentation with currently illegal drugs, as opposed to alcohol and tobacco dealt with above, has been a postwar phenomenon, and the efforts of successive editions of this Handbook to bring itself up to date show how rapidly the situation alters. This is due to several factors, including the changing availability of drugs, the fickleness of adolescent fashion and the varying impact of the world drug problem on schoolchildren. The current high cost of lysergide and opiates has fortunately led to their being used much less by schoolchildren, while their place as a major provoker of anxiety in school authorities has been taken by inhaled solvents. This is itself only the resurgence of a very ancient form of drug abuse.

As with alcohol, a distinction needs to be made between the physical, social and legal effects of single episodes of drug abuse, and the risk of dependence. The World Health Organisation definition of dependence[23], agreed in 1969, is still useful:

'A state, psychic and sometimes also physical, resulting from the interaction between a living organism and a drug, characterized by behavioural and other responses that always include a compulsion to take the drug on a continuous or periodic basis in order to experience a psychic effect, and sometimes to avoid the discomfort of its absence. Tolerance may or may not be present. A person may be dependent on more than one drug'.

There is now less confidence in distinguishing between psychic and physical dependence and between so-called hard and soft drugs. The groups of drugs which are commonly misused are as follows.

Narcotics

These are the opium derivates, diamorphine and morphine, and the synthetic narcotics, such as pethidine, dipipanone and methadone. They are the most dangerous drugs of addiction, particularly when administered intravenously, leading to tolerance (the need for ever-increasing dosage) and severe withdrawal symptoms. Some of those attracted to the narcotic way of life have profound personality disorders. There is a significant mortality rate from overdose, personal neglect and hepatitis.

Stimulants

Abuse of amphetamine and methylphenidate for their stimulant properties has diminished as more responsible prescribing has reduced their availability. On the other hand, cocaine, sniffed or taken by mouth, has increased in popularity among certain coteries which are able to afford the high price.

Hypnotics

The main group of hypnotics which has been widely abused is the barbiturates: they can cause physical dependence and withdrawal symptoms which include convulsions. The practice of extracting the powder from capsules, mixing it with water, and injecting intravenously was a particularly dangerous one. As in the case of amphetamines, the supply of barbiturates for abuse is diminishing as safer hypnotics are replacing them for legitimate medical needs.

Hallucinogens

This is the group of illegal drugs which has been most widely used in schools and society at large. Unlike the previous categories, the hallucinogens have no significant medical use, although cannabis has been used in the past as a sedative.

Cannabis is the most widely used hallucinogen, and remains illegal under Class B of the Misuse of Drugs Act, 1971, although penalties for its possession are generally much less severe now than in the past. It is a complex substance derived from the Indian hemp plant *Cannabis sativa:* the active ingredients are tetrahydrocannabinols which are fat-soluble and therefore very slowly eliminated from the body. Marijuana is made from the dried flowering tops of the plant, and is smoked mixed with tobacco. The resin can also be smoked, but is increasingly taken by mouth in various forms.

Cannabis is the most controversial of all drugs. By many it is used instead of alcohol to produce a pleasant feeling of relaxation. This is a group rather than an individual activity, an aid to social pleasure given added glamour because it is controversial and illegal. Its effects include euphoria, loquaciousness and excessive laughter, leading to confusion of identity, place and time, and later to hallucinations. The appearance of the patient under the effects of cannabis is that of apparent drunkenness, with bloodshot eyes, dry mouth, flushed face and excessive sleepiness. The variation of effect on individuals is widely held to be greater than with other drugs. Unlike alcohol it cannot be measured in body fluids, and as it undoubtedly affects driving skills this is one of the strongest arguments against removing it from the constraints of the Misuse of Drugs Act.

Lysergide (lysergic acid diethylamide, or LSD) is a much more potent and dangerous hallucinogen, which is easily synthesized, and was very widely available until the major UK source was tracked down by the police in the late 1970s. Its dose is hard to control, and many users have suffered the effects of horrifying hallucinations and the 'flashbacks' which can occur long after taking the drug. Lysergide is a colourless, tasteless liquid which is usually impregnated as a microdot on to small pieces of paper. It is included with the opiates in Class A of the Dangerous Drugs Act. It is making a reappearance in the United Kingdom, but its price is high.

Other hallucinogens not currently prevalent include mescaline, the description of which by Alduous Huxley [24] played a part in the explosion of drug experimentation in the 1960s.

Psilocybine is an hallucinogen derived from the common 'liberty cap' mushroom *(Psilocybe semilanceata)* which grows in the UK in the autumn. It has recently come to the attention of young people who have nicknamed it 'magic mushroom', and cases of hallucinations from its ingestion are becoming more common[25]. Psilocybine is not destroyed by heat, so it can be taken in a 'mushroom stew'. The effects include dilated pupils, tachycardia, euphoria, hallucinations and nausea. At present there is no law covering psilocybine, but the mushrooms constitute a definite risk, both from the direct effect of the hallucinations and from the possibility of people consuming poisonous fungi by mistake.

Glues and solvents

The arrival in the United Kingdom in the early 1970s of the solvent abuse craze which was already well established in the USA has brought with it a corresponding growth in the medical literature, critically reviewed by Black[26].

A variety of household solvents, including modelling glues, lighter fuel, nail-polish removers, trichlorethylene, paint thinners, erasing fluids and marking pencils, are used by pouring or squeezing the substance on to a rag or into a small bag and inhaling. The effects are mild intoxication and disinhibition, which may progress to hallucination, drowsiness and unconsciousness. The main risks are from inhalation of vomit and asphyxia from plastic bags adhering to the face, and these have probably accounted for most of the 45 deaths reported over a 7 year period in the United Kingdom[27].

As with many kinds of drug abuse, solvent abuse appears to be a comparatively harmless form of experimentation in the great majority, for whom it is a cheap alternative to alcohol. In a smaller group of disturbed adolescents, however, it becomes a habitual and dangerous form of deviant behaviour. There is some justification for the belief [28] that it is a passing fashion which will in due course be replaced by something else. Meanwhile, school authorities would be well advised to discourage the practice as unsensationally as possible.

Sex

Before addressing the 'problems' of sex in the adolescent it is chastening for school doctors to recall how misleading the pronouncements of some of our forebears have been. Whatever his personal opinions the school doctor must accept the changes in sexual attitudes and behaviour revealed in several studies reviewed by Rutter[9] who concludes, 'Clearly, premarital sex has now become the normal pattern. On the other hand, for many young people the sexual experience has only been with the person they subsequently married'. It is therefore muddled thinking to equate premarital sex with promiscuity. Nevertheless, the consequences of the changes in adolescent sexual behaviour have many medical implications, such as the correlation between early sexual debut and the subsequent development of cervical carcinoma.

Contraception

Although there has been a considerable increase in the use of effective methods of contraception among adolescents, it is clear that an alarmingly large number fail to employ them. There can be no doubt that contraception should be part of the curriculum of all schoolchildren: but at what age and in what manner it should be introduced is a matter for continuing debate. The issue which causes most difficulty to school doctors is the prescription of the contraceptive pill, as it can raise ethical as well as medical difficulties. Although a doctor's first duty is to his patient, the school doctor, by virtue of his appointment, also has an obligation to the school and to the parents. His best course therefore is to try to enlist their cooperation via the girl herself. In the case of prescribing contraceptives, this means that where there seems a real need the situation should be explained to the girl and help offered, if possible with the agreement of her parents. However, the overriding need to protect girls from unwanted pregnancy cannot be overstressed – a pregnancy which has to be terminated must be avoided at almost any cost because, however carefully and skilfully the operation is done, there is a small risk of subsequent infertility which can cause very bitter unhappiness in later life.

The doctor who prescribes contraceptives may be accused of implicitly encouraging the girl to have sexual intercourse. This ignores the fact that nearly half of the 16–19-year-olds interviewed by Farrell and Kellaher[29] had not used any contraceptive method during their first sexual experience, and that the great majority of girls approaching doctors for contraceptives are already at risk. Pupils over 16 are entitled to total confidentiality from their doctors, and this cannot be set aside for the sake of the school. Nevertheless, the implications within the school setting as well as for the individual should be reviewed in the counselling interview which should follow the request. The position with patients under 16 is less well defined, and the doctor must exercise the greatest care and judgement.

The advice of the General Medical Council[30] is as follows:

'Where a minor requests treatment concerning a pregnancy or contraceptive advice, the doctor should particularly have in mind the need to avoid impairing parental responsibility or family stability. The doctor should assess the patient's degree of parental dependence and seek to persuade the patient to involve the parents (or guardian or other person *in loco parentis*) from the earliest stage of consultation. If the patient refuses to allow a parent to be told, the doctor must observe the rule of professional secrecy in his management of the case'.

Some school doctors will only prescribe contraceptives to girls who obtain written parental permission, but this safeguard for the doctor has to be balanced against the fact that it is seldom difficult for the girl to obtain contraceptives without the parents' or doctors' knowledge. The doctor may have difficulty in keeping the respect of both the school authorities and his patients in this understandably sensitive area, but must do his best by displaying an openness and integrity while refusing to bend to pressure to break medical confidentiality.

Issues which are of concern to the doctor in prescribing contraceptives for pupils include the long-term risks of early sexual debut, the risk of venereal disease and the strain on an adolescent who, while apparently ready for the physical aspect of sexual experience, may be too immature to cope with the emotional commitment involved. The doctor will be aware of the greater permanence looked for by the female partner than the male for whom sexual adventure carries less commitment. He will also be concerned about the group of adolescent girls in whom a childhood deprived of love may lead to an emotional poverty compensated for by sexual promiscuity.

Pregnancy and termination

Pregnancy in young schoolgirls carries a higher than average risk of complications, including stillbirth, premature birth and low birth-weight babies. When a pregnancy is discovered, efforts should be made to obtain the parents' understanding and help, although the girl's agreement should be obtained first. Each situation has to be judged on its merits, but in many cases termination can be justified in the present climate of opinion and the earlier this is done the less the risk. The doctor's full and immediate help is therefore of great importance. Section 1(a) of the Abortion Act 1967 provides that no offence is caused when two medical practitioners are of the opinion formed in good faith that 'the continuation of the pregnancy would involve . . . . . . injury to the physical or mental health of the pregnant woman'.

Court[31] emphasized the importance of skilled counselling and the opportunity for discussion before any decision is taken, including the participation wherever possible of the whole family and particularly the boyfriend.

Sexually transmitted diseases

There has been a steady increase in the incidence of sexually trans-mitted diseases among adolescents, and teaching on the subject is an essential part of any health education programme. Clinical aspects are dealt with in Chapter 9 (p. 170).

Masturbation

Masturbation is now universally regarded as a normal and harmless activity and seldom causes the anxiety and guilt which were so common in the past.

Sexual offences

The school doctor may be consulted when a pupil is the victim of a sexual offence, such as indecent exposure, indecent assault, rape, buggery, bestiality, acts of gross indecency between men, unlawful sexual intercourse and incest. Rape can vary from a violent 'gang bang' causing physical harm to sexual intercourse between two young people when the offender thought that consent was being given. Incest, which is now known to be much commoner than once thought, can vary from sexual intercourse forced upon an unwilling daughter by a violent father to intercourse between a father and daughter in circumstances in which the wife colludes.

Consent to sexual intercourse is invalid if the girl is under the age of 16 years. It is defence for an accused man under 24 if he genuinely believes the girl to have been 16 or over, but the plea operates only once.

A doctor having knowledge of a sexual offence has the same responsibility as in the case of any other kind of offence, but should bear in mind that the law takes a particularly serious view of sexual offences against children and young persons. The protection of other vulnerable youngsters who may become victims is an important factor, but the doctor's responsibility to the patient is paramount. When a sexual offence such as rape or indecent assault is alleged, early detailed examination is necessary for forensic reasons. If possible this should be entrusted to an experienced police surgeon as special skills are involved.

Education on sex and drugs

Most of the matters dealt with in this chapter should be part of a child's health education. Doctors may be asked to advise or participate, but it must be recognized that health education is increasingly a professional skill of teachers, many of whom are specially qualified in the subject. The doctor may well contribute so long as his skills of communication match his professional knowledge. The advice of the Department of Education and Science[32] to those approaching sex education is worth quoting in full:

'Those who embark on a deliberate policy of sex education and education in personal relationships in schools of all types are faced with the following questions:

(1) Why? What are the aims, both short-term and long-term? This is the most difficult question of all but it must be answered before going on.

(2) Who should be responsible for the teaching? Many boys and girls are embarrassed by 'trendy' teachers, and all are

immediately aware of hypocrisy and dishonesty in adults, and many teachers are embarrassed by the task.

(3) What underlying value judgements are assumed? These must be identified and defended.

(4) What are we going to teach? A foundation of biological knowledge? If so, will it include information about family planning, contraception, venereal diseases, and sexual deviations?

(5) At what stages in school life will the teaching be attempted, and why?

(6) What methods of teaching will be adopted? Exposition, discussion, individual counselling, individualized learning (tapes, projected material, books, etc. for private study)?

(7) To what extent are the influences of the whole curriculum and the life of the school taken into account? This is a very important question because discussion of sexual matters can so easily be overemphasized.

(8) How does the school co-operate with parents and others responsible for the children?

There are no standard answers to these questions applicable to all types of school'.

Even more teasing philosophical questions are posed by education on drug abuse. Blum[33] has confirmed the suspicion that education may actually increase drug experimentation, and the Institute for the Study of Drug Dependence caused controversy by suggesting that it might be better to teach schoolchildren how to practise glue sniffing more safely than to drive the habit underground by a totally prohibitive attitude[34].

References

1. Sheridan, M. D. (1975). *The Developmental Progress of Infants and Young Children*. 3rd Edn. DHSS Report No. 102. (London: HMSO)
2. Tanner, J. M. (1978). *Education and Physical Growth*. 2nd Edn. (London: Hodder and Stoughton)
3. Clow, A. E. S. (1923). The effects of physical exercise and menstruation. *J. Sch. Hyg. Phys. Educ.* 15, 64
4. Eykyn, S. J. (1982). Toxic shock syndrome: some answers but questions remain. *Br. Med J.*, 284, 1585
5. Freud, A. (1958). Adolescence. *Psychoanalyt. Study Child,* 13, 255

6. Erikson, E. H. (1955). The problem of ego identity. *J. Am. Psychoanal. Assoc.*, 4, 56
7. Erikson, E. H. (1977). *Childhood and Society.* (St Albans: Triad/Paladin)
8. Miller, D. (1969). *The Age Between.* p. 135 (London: Cornmarket-Hutchinson)
9. Rutter, M. (1979). *Changing Youth in a Changing Society.* (London: The Nuffield Provincial Hospitals Trust)
10. Hadfield, J. A. (1962). *Childhood and Adolescence.* p. 205. (Harmondsworth: Penguin Books)
11. Dally, P. and Gomez, J. (1980). *Obesity and Anorexia Nervosa.* p. 76. (London: Faber and Faber)
12. Crisp, A. H. (1977). The differential diagnosis of anorexia nervosa. *Proc. R. Soc. Med.,* 70, 686
13. Lacy, J. H. (1976). Anorexia nervosa. *Nursing Times,* 72, 407
14. Olweus, D. (1978). *Aggression in Schools – Bullies and Whipping Boys.* (New York: Hemisphere Publishing Corporation)
15. Orton, W. J. (1982). Mobbing. *Publ. Hlth.,* 96, 172
16. Hemming, J. (1983). Motivation for violence among adolescents. Presented at a Medical Officers of Schools Association Symposium on Mobbing, May 20, 1982. *Publ. Hlth.,* 97, 324.
17. Royal College of Psychiatrists (1979). *Alcohol and Alcoholism.* The Report of a Special Committee. (London: Tavistock Publications)
18. Dobbs, J. and Marsh, A. (1983) *Smoking among Secondary School Children.* (London: HMSO)
19. McKennell, A. C. and Thomas, R. K. (1967). *Adults' and Adolescents' Smoking Habits and Attitudes.* Government Social Survey. (London: HMSO)
20. Bynner, J. M. (1969). *The Young Smoker.* Government Social Survey. (London: HMSO)
21. Bewley, B. R., Day I, and Ide, L. (1974). *Smoking by Children in Great Britain.* (London: Medical Research Council)
22. Edwards, G. (1971). *Unreason in an Age of Reason.* (London: Royal Society of Medicine)
23. World Health Organization (1969). WHO Expert Committee on Drug Dependence. Sixteenth Report. *Tech. Rep. Series No. 407.*
24. Huxley, A. (1954). *The Doors of Perception.* (London: Chatto & Windus)
25. Young, R. E., Milroy, R., Hutchinson, S. and Kesson, C. M. (1982). The rising price of mushrooms. *Lancet,* 1, 213
26. Black, D. (1982). Glue sniffing. *Arch. Dis. Child.,* 57, 893
27. Watson, J. M. (1979). Morbidity and mortality statistics on solvent abuse. *Med. Sci. Law,* 19, 246
28. Freeston, U. (1983). Glue sniffer's guide. *Update,* 26, 1921
29. Farrell, C. and Kellaher, L. (1978). *My Mother Said: The Way Young People Learn about Sex and Birth Control.* (London: Routledge and Kegan Paul)
30. General Medical Council (1983). *Professional Conduct and Discipline: Fitness to Practise* (London: GMC)
31. Cmnd. 6684 (1976). *Fit for the Future.* Vol. 1. The Report of the Committee on Child Health Services. p. 168. (London: HMSO)
32. Department of Education and Science (1977). *Health Education in Schools.* (London: HMSO)
33. Blum, R. H. (1976). *Drug Education: Results and Recommendations.* (Lexington, Mass.: Lexington Books)
34. Institute for the Study of Drug Dependence (1980). *Teaching about a Volatile Situation.* (London: ISDD)

CHAPTER 5

SOME MEDICAL PROBLEMS OF CHILDHOOD AND ADOLESCENCE

Acne vulgaris

This is the commonest skin condition of adolescence, and the school doctor should not underestimate its importance to many of those who suffer from it. It is very amenable to treatment, but this requires understanding and perseverance.

An essential factor in acne is excessive sebum production by the sebaceous glands which are sensitive to androgens, although the precise mechanism is not clear. The pilosebaceous ducts become blocked with keratin, forming blackheads, and these may in turn become colonized with bacteria which produce inflammation.

Local treatment

There have been considerable advances in topical preparations since the last edition of the Handbook. Benzoyl peroxide is most effective, and is available as a gel, cream or lotion in various bases in concentrations of 2.5%, 5% and 10%. Tretinoin, a vitamin A derivative, acts by loosening the keratin plug, and is particularly useful for the treatment of multiple comedones, although it can cause redness and peeling of the skin.

Antibiotic treatment

Antibiotics are highly effective and without risk if used in therapeutic doses for as long as the condition persists. They should be used in all cases of pustular acne causing any embarrassment or distress to the sufferer. Oxytetracycline is the antibiotic of choice and, of the minority who do not respond, nearly all do so to co-trimoxazole or erythromycin. It is usual to start with one tablet (250 mg of oxytet-racycline and erythromycin, 480 mg of co-trimoxazole) two or three times a day. The therapeutic response may not occur for a month or more, after which the dose can usually be reduced. Tetracyclines are poorly absorbed if taken with food or milk, and for optimum effect should be taken about 30 minutes before meals. The treatment must continue for several months at least, and is often needed for two or three years.

Hormone treatment

In intractable cases in girls, oral contraceptives containing 50 μg of ethinyloestradiol may be effective. Ethinyloestradiol can be combined with the antiandrogen cyproterone acetate in a single tablet, but this should be reserved for the most difficult cases when other methods have been fully tried, and is contraindicated in pregnancy.

Isotretinoin

Oral isotretinoin holds great promise, but has potentially serious side-effects, and can only be prescribed at present by dermatologists.

Diet

Although there is no objective evidence for the value of dietary measures, some patients insist that their acne improves if they avoid chocolate and reduce their carbohydrate intake.

Allergic conditions

The allergies which most commonly cause problems amongst schoolchildren are hay fever, allergic rhinitis and asthma.

Hay fever causes disproportionate concern as the pollen season often coincides with public examinations, but recent advances have greatly improved the doctor's ability to relieve symptoms. To reduce contact with pollen, the patient should keep his bedroom window closed during the day and wear glasses out of doors during the hay fever season. Antihistamines give good symptomatic relief in many patients, but the response in terms of effectiveness and sedative side-effects is individually determined. The majority of children and adolescents do not suffer from drowsiness when taking chlorpheniramine maleate, which may conveniently be given in a sustained-release tablet twice a day. When sedation does occur, the more expensive terfenadine may be substituted. When eye irritation is troublesome, antihistamine (antazoline with xylometazoline), cromoglycate or steroid eye drops may be used, provided care is taken in the case of steroid drops to exclude the possibility of *Herpes simplex* infection which may lead to dentritic ulcers. Rhinitis may be controlled by local cromoglycate or corticosteroid nasal sprays. With these locally-acting agents available, oral and parenteral steroid will seldom be needed. Depot injections of steroid carry a greater risk of adrenocortical suppression than oral prednisolone and should be used with caution. They can, nevertheless, be dramatically effective in a crisis (such as severe symptoms presenting in the week of an examination).

Allergic rhinitis can cause a lot of misery and may need to be treated in collaboration with an ear, nose and throat surgeon. Antihistamines, cromoglycate and local corticosteroids can be helpful. If skin tests are carried out, the allergen will often prove to be the house dust mite, which is as prevalent in boarding school dormitories as in private houses. Its precise role in causing symptoms remains uncertain, and it is impossible to exclude it completely from the environment. Nevertheless, removal of feather bedding and substitution of foam rubber for conventional pillows can be very effective. Hyposensitizing injections are seldom rewarding.

Asthma

The life of the asthmatic schoolchild in the 1980s is much easier than in the past, thanks to a better understanding of the condition by doctors and lay people alike, and a greatly improved range of preventive and symptom-controlling treatment. The principal aim of management of the asthmatic pupil must be to enable him to lead a normal school life, and all but the most severely affected should be able to do so. The school doctor must be able to provide rapid and effective action in an asthmatic attack, while seeing that when the patient is well he has as little anxiety and special care as possible.

Scadding[1] defines asthma as 'a disease characterized by wide variations over short periods of time in resistance to flow in intrapulmonary airways'. In most cases in children asthma is extrinsic, due to hypersensitivity to airborne allergens such as pollens and the faeces of the house dust mite. Their wheezing may be triggered off by exercise, cold air, other people's tobacco smoke, and, less frequently than is often supposed, by viral respiratory infections. A chronic nocturnal cough is often a symptom of asthma, and the formerly popular diagnosis of 'wheezy bronchitis' should be abandoned in favour of asthma, which is invariably the correct diagnosis. There is evidence [2] that some general practitioners are still preoccupied with infection as a principal cause of respiratory symptoms in childhood. Emotion is not a cause of asthma, although it may precipitate an attack in an asthmatic subject. It needs to be understood by doctors, nurses and teachers that asthma is neither a symptom of respiratory infection nor a psychosomatic condition. This means that some methods of treatment which were commonly used in the past should be abandoned. Sedatives and tranquillizers can depress the respiratory centre and may therefore be dangerous as well as inappropriate, while antibiotics are seldom indicated, and should only be considered by the doctor after treatment to deal with the bronchospasm has been instituted.

The essential tool in the assessment of asthma is the peak flow meter. It provides an accurate measurement of the degree of airway obstruction which is much more reliable than the patient's own assessment of the severity of his symptoms or the sounds heard through the stethoscope.

A small proportion, about 2.5%, of asthmatic children have chronic asthma with daily wheezing, which may be associated with growth failure and pigeon chest. These require the most intensive long-term therapy: some can cope in the normal school environment, but some need to be in special schools.

Treatment in occasional asthma

The child who has occasional attacks is best treated with a selective bronchodilator such as salbutamol or terbutaline in a pressurized aerosol inhaler. It is essential to instruct the patient carefully in its use and ensure that the technique has been mastered. For those who have difficulty with aerosol inhalers, dried powder inhalers may be managed more easily. The inhaler has to be readily available for use, and this can present management difficulties. For younger children, teachers may look after the inhaler provided its purpose has been explained, but in most cases it is sensible to allow the pupil to keep the aerosol in a pocket; in practice very few patients overuse their inhalers.

Attacks of exertional asthma can often be prevented by using the inhaler before games.

There is no place for the use of antihistamines, either in tablets or cough mixture form, as they have no effect on asthma.

Treatment of more severe and more continuous asthma

The choice of long-term treatment needs to be fully discussed with the patient and the parents. Sustained release aminophylline or theophylline preparations are sometimes effective. If these or salbutamol or terbutaline in a regular dose of 2 puffs, 4 times a day, fail to control the asthma, regular cromoglycate at the same intervals may do so: it can be given either as spincaps in a rotahaler or as an aerosol inhaler; the preparation combined with isoprenaline should never be prescribed. If cromoglycate is ineffective, inhaled beclomethasone or betamethosone should be given, again in a dose of 2 puffs, 4 times a day, initially: it may later be possible to control symptoms with a less frequent dose. It is unnecessary to give cromoglycate simultaneously: the cromoglycate should be withdrawn when the patient starts on inhaled steroids.

If symptoms deteriorate despite the full use of inhaled steroids, oral steroids may be needed, either as short courses of fairly large doses, or on a regular basis, adjusted to the minimum dose which will control symptoms. Some patients can be maintained on an alternate day dose, and this may reduce the risk of side-effects including growth retardation.

Severe asthma

Medical, nursing and ancillary staff must be able to recognize the signs of severe, dangerous asthma, remembering the continuing incidence of sudden unexpected death. In nearly every case this is found to be due to underestimation of the severity of the attack and consequent undertreatment. Wheeze may be absent in severe cases, so the use of the peak flow meter is essential. Cyanosis, inappropriate tachycardia, pulsus paradoxus, speech impairment and confusion are all serious prognostic signs, and early intervention is necessary. An increasing number of hospitals have arrangements for immediate admission of asthmatics, sometimes by self-referral. However, many children respond rapidly to bronchodilators such as salbutamol by nebulizer. Effective nebulizers using a footpump are inexpensive, and should be part of the equipment of every school sanatorium. If the nebulizer does not bring immediate improvement intravenous steroids must be given in a large dose: at least 200 mg of hydrocortisone – some would say as much as 500 mg. Sedation should never be given, and admission to hospital should not be delayed.

Diabetes mellitus

Most diabetics can cope well with school, including boarding school, and the doctor can play an important part in holding the balance between the anxiety of the parents, the fears of the school and the needs of the diabetic child. The routine of the school day can be a useful framework for establishing a balance between meals, insulin and activity. The school has to understand that the diabetic will need regular snacks between meals at times when other pupils may not be allowed to eat. He will also need snacks, in the form of chocolate, sweets, sugar or crisps, before unusual activity such as an examination or sport. On the other hand, the diabetic pupil may need to avoid sweets and puddings at main meals, substituting fresh fruit if possible.

Management is easiest when the child has learned to give his own insulin injection, and when diet is not too rigidly controlled. The pupil should monitor his own urine or blood sugar: this is comparatively simple with the help of diagnostic strips which can be held in the urine stream and automated blood sugar testing kits. Fellow pupils and staff should have the condition explained to them unsensationally, including the signs of hypoglycaemic attacks. Provided the school is aware of his condition, the diabetic can take part in all sports, including swimming.

Those in charge should tactfully watch to see that he remembers to have a snack before swimming, for example, and to provide help quickly if difficulties should arise. Everyone should know where the child or teacher keeps the emergency sugar supply: 6 dextrosol sweets will be needed for a hypoglycaemic attack. In the case of hypoglycaemic coma, an injection of glucagon, 1 mg intramuscularly or subcutaneously in the deltoid region or front of the thigh, can prevent prolonged unconsciousness and a trip to hospital. Prepacked ampoules are easy to use, and teachers and older pupils are often prepared to learn how to give them if a pupil is known to be liable to such attacks.

The care and storage of syringes can be a problem in boarding schools. It is now accepted that disposable syringes and needles can be used many times provided they are stored dry in a refrigerator and handled only by the patient.

The doctor must be prepared for the patient to rebel against the discipline of injections and diet at some time during adolescence, and should take into account that too authoritarian a response is counter-productive. Similarly, parents have to steer a course between being uninterested and obsessional. The diabetic, who has to cope with the problems of adolescence aggravated by the diabetes, has to be helped to progress from childhood to adulthood as if he were without the disease. Careers advisers need to be informed about the difficulties diabetics may experience in getting work. Careers in which a hypoglycaemic attack could be dangerous must be avoided. Diabetics cannot, for example, hold a heavy goods vehicle or public service vehicle licence.

Address

British Diabetic Association,
10 Queen Anne Street,
London W1M 0BD
(Telephone: 01-323 1531)

Enuresis and soiling

90% of children are dry by the age of 5 years and 95% by the age of 8 years. A small proportion continue to have nocturnal enuresis into their teens and early adult life. The condition tends to occur in families, which lends support to the belief that primary enuresis is due to late maturation of bladder control. Emotional factors may complicate the management of primary enuresis. Physical causes such as urinary infection need to be excluded, but in the majority of cases none are found and the condition is properly regarded as a behaviour disorder.

In the management of the younger child with primary nocturnal enuresis, it is sometimes effective to ask the child to devise a calendar in which dry nights are rewarded with a star. Failing this, the enuresis alarm (bell and pad) provides the best hope of success[3]. Another form of treatment which is often successful is imipramine, although its mode of action is uncertain. The normal dose is 25–50 mg at night, but it is inadvisable to use it for more than a few months. Unfortunately, relapse often occurs after the drug is withdrawn, but it can be a very useful way of taking the heat out of the situation at boarding school.

Faecal soiling may be due simply to chronic constipation leading to overflow incontinence. The constipation may be due to Hirschsprung's disease, and children with prolonged symptoms should be referred for investigation. Simple constipation may need to be treated with laxatives and suppositories to clear the rectum followed by bowel training under careful supervision. Soiling may also occur in association with symptoms of a serious emotional upset. In these cases it is much more difficult to control. Care must be taken not to add to the emotional difficulties by the excessive use of laxatives, suppositories or enemata. It should be emphasized to the school staff that a punitive attitude is harmful in all cases of enuresis and faecal soiling.

Epilepsy

In the care of the epileptic schoolchild, the school doctor must be prepared not only to supervise the drug regime, but to help the patient to cope optimistically with the disability, participate as fully as possible in school life, and prepare for a suitable occupation. The aim of drug therapy is to find a dose of a single drug which will control attacks without giving rise to side-effects. In grand mal, temporal lobe and focal epilepsy carbamazepine is the first choice of most physicians, followed by phenobarbitone and phenytoin. Combinations of drugs are seldom necessary, and should be avoided if possible. In petit mal, ethosuximide or sodium valproate are used.

The single attack presents a problem of management, in which the degree of certainty of diagnosis, family history, presence or absence of head injury and EEG result will all help in the decision whether to treat the patient or not. Status epilepticus is an emergency requiring urgent hospitalization after giving diazepam 0.3 mg/kg, up to a maximum of 10 mg, intravenously over 2–3 minutes.

Adolescents in particular have to make personal adjustments to their epilepsy, and require regular, sympathetic and firm management. They must be advised to avoid the factors which precipitate attacks, including irregular hours and alcohol excess. At school they should be encouraged to lead as active a life as possible, including virtually all sports. Very few restrictions are necessary. Unless the epileptic always has an aura, he should not swim alone or climb in the gymnasium. When a pupil with epilepsy participates in group swimming at school there should be a well-informed adult available on the bath side who knows that the child has epilepsy and can carry out resuscitation if a convulsion should occur. Mountain climbing is not advisable, but a decision on cycling must depend on the frequency of attacks and volume of traffic on the road to be travelled on.

Epileptics will need careers guidance as some occupations, such as the police and armed forces, are closed to them. They will not be able to drive public service or heavy goods vehicles, but a driving licence to drive a private car may be granted after two years' freedom from waking attacks.

Address

British Epilepsy Association, Crowthorne House,
Bigshotte, New Wokingham Road, Wokingham, Berkshire.
(Telephone: 0734 3122).

Headaches and migraine

In the differential diagnosis of headaches, organic causes are the rarest but potentially the most serious. They include meningitis, encephalitis, tumours, and headache due to solvent abuse and lead encephalopathy. The commonest type of headache is tension headache, which occurs every day in the majority of sufferers. This helps to distinguish tension headaches from migraine, which never occurs as often.

The onset of migraine is usually before the age of 20. Sparks [4] found an incidence of 3.37% among 12 543 boys and 2.5% among 3 242 girls aged 10–18 years in a survey of MOSA schoolchildren. The figures for boys are very close to those of Bille [5] in Uppsala, but in common with others Bille found a higher rate (4.41%) among girls aged 7–15. The different results of the two surveys may perhaps be explained by Bille's observation that remission commonly occurs between the ages of 9 and 16 years.

In classical migraine, the headache is usually described as a severe pain, which is unilateral (the 'hemicrania' which gives migraine its name). It is accompanied by nausea, vomiting and focal symptoms. These are usually sensory in the form of visual disturbances – flashing lights, fortification spectra and distorted vision – but they may also take the form of motor disturbances, aphasia and mood change. The attack usually ends with the patient falling asleep. Variations include non-classical migraine, in which there are no focal symptoms, and hemiplegic migraine. There is often a family history of migraine – and occasionally a history of travel sickness.

The causes include dietary (food and also starvation), endocrine, psychological, hereditary and allergic. The commonest food implicated is chocolate, followed by cheese, citrus fruits and alcohol in descending order of importance. The best advice on diet is to avoid only things which are known to upset the patient. The treatment of an attack consists of rest, an antiemetic (such as metoclopramide, 5 mg for 10-year-olds, 10 mg for adults) and an analgesic (aspirin or paracetamol) given 10 minutes after the antiemetic. Some patients get extrapyramidal reactions to metoclopramide, but these disappear spontaneously. Ergotamine is very rarely necessary and poisoning, with symptoms confusingly similar to migraine, readily occurs.

Address

British Migraine Association,
178a High Road, Byfleet,
Weybridge, Surrey, KT14 7ED.
(Telephone: 0932 352468).

Orthopaedic problems

There are two sites in which non-traumatic orthopaedic conditions are particularly likely to present in the school years, the back and the hip.

Scoliosis

Idiopathic adolescent scoliosis is a condition which has been neglected in the past. The cause is unknown, and 90% of cases occur in girls. The painless lateral deviation of the spinal column progresses quickly at the time of the adolescent growth spurt, and early detection is essential if treatment is to be instituted before skeletal growth is over. A minor degree of scoliosis can be found in 5% of adolescent girls, but only 0.2% develop progressive curvature which requires treatment.

A screening programme in 10–15-year-old children is essential for the prevention of permanent deformity. The forward bending test should therefore be a part of every school medical examination (including the school entry examination, to detect infantile and juvenile scoliosis) (Chapter 2, p. 26). If a child shows asymmetry of the rib cage when bending forward, she should be followed up for signs of increase in the asymmetry. The difficulty of such a programme lies in deciding at what point a child should be referred to an orthopaedic clinic for examination and X-rays. If the curvature of the spine reaches 20°, treatment with a brace may be instituted, and if it progresses to 50° operation is usually advisable. There is no evidence that exercises or physiotherapy have any effect on the progress of the condition.

The hip

The purpose of including the hip in this section is to remind school doctors and nurses of the care needed in assessing symptoms which may arise in the hip joint. The common symptoms, which may appear trivial, are limp and pain, and they may deceptively be referred to the knee.

Congenital dislocation should be detected in infancy, but David *et al.*[6] showed how frequently the diagnosis is made late, often well into the nursery school age group. Limping was the commonest presenting symptom. Perthe's disease (osteochondritis of the femoral capital epiphysis) presents in the primary school age group, as does transient arthritis which has similar symptoms. X-rays are essential in the differential diagnosis.

A pitfall in the adolescent is slipped femoral epiphysis, which causes gradual onset of pain and limp. Half the cases occur in the characteristic 'fat-boy-of Dickens' type, the others in boys and girls of normal build. Complications due to avascular necrosis and later osteoarthritis are common, so early diagnosis and referral are imperative. Slipped epiphysis should be suspected in every adolescent who complains of pain in the hip or knee; if the symptom persists a lateral X-ray of the hip is advisable.

Menstrual and gynaecological problems

Dysmenorrhoea

This is a common and important problem in school medicine. A distinction must be made from the mild malaise, often with low backache, which is quite common and should be ignored by the girls as far as possible. They should be encouraged to continue with their normal sporting activities. Unfortunately, menstruation is liable to be used as an excuse by those who do not relish these active pursuits, whereas those who are good at sport will usually play matches and compete in athletics regardless. Excuses from games on account of menstruation therefore should not be encouraged.

There is, however, a different condition which affects many girls occasionally but a few often – primary spasmodic dysmenorrhoea, which has a very characteristic pattern. It occurs just before or in the early part of the flow and the pain is in the centre of the lower abdomen, often radiating down the thighs. It can be very severe indeed and faintness or vomiting are sometimes associated. It may be completely incapacitating while it lasts, but as this is seldom more than a few hours, half a day away from school is usually all that is needed. Many cases, but not all, are helped considerably by drugs with an inhibiting effect on prostaglandin synthetase. Aspirin is one of these, but mefenamic acid, flurbiprofen and similar drugs are more potent. Indomethacin suppositories are valuable where vomiting is a problem. It cannot be stressed too strongly that no addictive drug must ever be given for this condition, tempting as it may often be to use morphine or pethidine. Bed with a hot water bottle is still a great comfort and often leads to sleep for a few hours with complete recovery on waking.

Another point must be made here – a girl's future can be in jeopardy if she is incapacitated by dysmenorrhoea on the day of an important examination or interview. Therefore, sufferers from this condition should be known to the doctor so that a reliable remedy is found for them well in advance. Dydrogesterone is prophylactic in some cases (possibly as many as 60%) so is worth a try in a dose of 10 mg twice daily from day 5 to day 25 of the menstrual month; it does not inhibit ovulation. As this type of dysmenorrhoea only occurs in ovulatory cycles a valuable and reliable remedy is to prevent ovulation using a low oestrogen contraceptive pill. Operative treatment for dysmenorrhoea is not recommended.

Mittelschmerz

Mid-cycle ovulation pain occurs at times in women and it is sometimes found in schoolgirls. No treatment except explanation and reassurance is usually required but the condition occasionally causes diagnostic problems. The pain may be referred to either iliac fossa or to the rectum. It varies in severity but seldom lasts more than 12–24 hours. Occasionally some vaginal bleeding occurs at this time but should not cause worry.

Menorrhagia

Heavy bleeding does sometimes occur in the early menstrual years and occasionally it is alarmingly severe. Rest and sedation may be all that is required, with iron to maintain the haemoglobin. Severer cases usually respond to hormone therapy. Progestogen can be given during the bleeding episode, e.g. norethisterone 15 mg daily, increasing, if necessary, to 10 mg 4 hourly until bleeding ceases. A smaller dose (5 mg b.d.) can then be continued until 3 weeks' freedom from bleeding has been achieved. It may be necessary to repeat the treatment for two or three months. In some cases oestrogen is more successful or a combined oestrogen–progestogen preparation.

Very occasionally, really dangerous bleeding can occur, requiring blood transfusion; although this is relatively rare, each case of prolonged bleeding should be under the doctor's close supervision, and gynaecological help sought before severe anaemia develops.

Irregularity

Irregularity of menstrual rhythm is common in the school age group. This should be accepted as part of the growing up process, and attempts to regulate the cycle by hormones should be avoided.

Amenorrhoea

Two problems may confront the school doctor: the girl who fails to commence menstruation with the rest of her age group – primary amenorrhoea; and the girl who starts and then stops – secondary amenorrhoea.

Although the menarche usually occurs between the ages of 11 and 13 years some girls start earlier and some as late as 16 or 17. The time to investigate the latter is when the girl or her parents are worried about it or at age 16. A useful clue is the onset of breast development. This usually precedes the menarche by a year or more. So if breast development has only recently been noted one should be optimistic that menstruation will start within 1–2 years, but if it has not begun by then further investigation should be instigated. Again, if there is no sign of breast development by 15 or 16 further investigation is advisable. Any sign of masculinity demands immediate and expert help, but fortunately this is very rare as doubtful sex is now recognized in the neonatal period and a decision made then.

Cryptomenorrhoea must also be remembered. In these cases there is normal breast development and periodic lower abdominal pain. Ultimately a lower abdominal swelling may appear but the obstruction must be relieved before then or the tubes may become damaged.

Secondary amenorrhoea is a big subject and cannot be fully dealt with here, but certain rules must be stressed. First, pregnancy must never be forgotten – a pelvic examination and an immunological pregnancy test are mandatory if there is the slightest doubt. If negative the girl should be checked again in 2–4 weeks, because tests are not always reliable and time can produce embarrassing evidence of a mistake! There are many other causes of secondary amenorrhoea, but emotional and environmental conditions explain most. Under-nutrition must be kept in mind as amenorrhoea may be a warning sign of anorexia nervosa. Diabetes, tuberculosis and thyroid dysfunction should be excluded if the amenorrhoea is persistent, and the possibility of the polycystic ovary syndrome must be remembered, especially if hirsutism and obesity are associated. It is usually sound to temporize with amenorrhoea for 6 months in the absence of any other abnormal signs. The production of a false period by hormone therapy is not advisable and can interfere with physiological recovery.

Premenstrual tension

This condition is in danger of being over-stressed with detriment to the rational attitude which must be adopted by women toward the cyclical variations of their physiology, as has already been discussed. It is probably true that most women are at their best just after menstruation and at their lowest in the few days before it. Fluid retention and a tendency to gut distension can be troublesome in the premenstrual week, resulting in a bloated feeling. This is more a complaint of the older age groups and should not be commonly encountered by the school doctor.

Vaginal discharge

This may occur at any age. In the very young it suggests an

infection and should be investigated as such, not forgetting however the possibility of threadworms, foreign bodies and trauma.

The prepubertal child of about 9–11 frequently goes through a phase of extra secretion sufficient to soil underclothes; this is normal and should be ignored unless it is causing soreness or irritation. Later, excessive secretion may occur from over-activity of the cervical glands (sometimes associated with a so-called congenital erosion). This again requires no treatment unless very excessive. The discharge is mucoid in these cases and may dry somewhat brown on the clothing, sometimes wrongly suggesting blood staining.

Infective discharges are not uncommon at school age. The most prevalent are moniliasis and *Trichomonas vaginalis* but gonorrhoea must never be forgotten. A vaginal swab should be despatched in transport medium, but unfortunately false negatives do occur especially with trichomonas infection. In the presence of marked irritation and a fairly copious discharge, an empirical course of metronidazole after taking a swab is a justifiable and reasonable course of action. Local treatment is only required for candida infections.

If venereal disease is suspected, or found, expert help should be sought without delay. Short intensive treatment can produce a rapid and complete cure. The forgotten tampon as an occasional cause of discharge has already been mentioned in Chapter 4 (p. 57).

The testis

Conditions of the testis commonly met with in school practice include the undescended testis, torsion of the testis, hydrocele, varicocele and trauma to the testis or scrotal contents, usually arising from games injury.

Torsion of the testis

Definition and cause

Rotation of the testis on its horizontal axis leads to twisting of the spermatic cord and impairment of the blood supply to the testis. Certain anatomical abnormalities, e.g. a horizontal lie of the testis, are thought to predispose to the occurrence. Torsion occurs most commonly in the prepubescent child and the adolescent. About half the cases occur during sleep, often in the early morning; the remainder during or shortly after severe physical exertion.

Diagnosis

The presenting symptom is pain, ranging from mild to excruciating, depending on the degree of torsion. The pain is usually scrotal, but may start in an iliac fossa, later radiating to the scrotum. There are no other early symptoms or signs except vomiting and shock in severe cases. Pyrexia is a later sign; dysuria is not a feature.

Sudden testicular pain in the schoolchild should alert all concerned to the possible diagnosis of torsion of the testis. Only when this has been excluded should alternative diagnoses, of which the acute orchitis of mumps (see p. 149) is the most likely, to be considered.

Early diagnosis is important. Unrelieved torsion of the spermatic cord leads sooner rather than later to destruction of the testis. Few testes survive a torsion of more than 12 hours.

Treatment

Relief of the condition in the early stages is simple. Manual rotation is effective, and can be performed without analgesia – on occasions, intravenous diazepam 10 mg may be required. If pain is severe, morphine or pethidine may be needed.

With the warm patient in the supine position the medical attendant gently rotates the testis using both hands. Correct detorsion brings immediate relief, incorrect rotation increases discomfort; the attendant in this event reverses the direction. The patient is witness to the success of the manoeuvre. Twists of less than 180° reduce themselves spontaneously.

The benefit of manipulative reduction is that the urgency is removed from the situation. Awareness of the condition, early diagnosis, prompt relief of the torsion, and bilateral orchidopexy should be accepted practice.

Torsion of the appendix testis (hydatid of Morgagni) occurs less commonly. The pain may be severe. If the diagnosis is definite no treatment is necessary – the appendix testis will eventually atrophy. If there is any doubt surgical exploration of the scrotum is advisable.

The undescended testis

In a full term male infant the testes should be in the scrotum at birth; a testis which has not attained this position is undescended. Scorer[7] reported the incidence of undescended testes at birth to be 4%.

Descent continues during the first year of life, and at 1 year of age the incidence of non-descent is 0.8%; this compares with the probable incidence in adulthood of 0.7%.

Clinically there are 5 groups.

(a)   The high scrotal testis, or incomplete descent. The testis never reaches the bottom of the scrotum, and always lies at a higher level than its larger (normal) fellow.

(b)   The intracanalicular testis. This is very difficult or impossible to feel. If palpable it can be manipulated downwards but always resumes its intracanalicular position.

(c)   The intra-abdominal testis which is impalpable, and often very difficult to find at operation. Occasionally a so-called intra-abdominal (missing) testis is diagnosed mistakenly for an unnoted perinatal torsion with subsequent atrophy of the testis.

(d)   The arrested (ectopic) testis. This is not an undescended testis but a maldescended one. The testis passes normally through the inguinal canal, fails to enter the scrotum, usually ascending obliquely upwards and laterally to lie in the superficial inguinal pouch. The importance of this sub-group is that the spermatic cord is of normal length, so that surgical intervention is more successful than in the treatment of the other groups.

(e)   There are other very rare sites where the testis is truly ectopic e.g. perineal.

The retractile testis is most often misdiagnosed in cases of bilateral non-descent. Only careful and, if necessary, repeated examination eliminates unnecessary surgical intervention.

The treatment of the undescended testis is surgical; current practice is to operate before the age of 6 years.

Hydrocele

Primary hydrocele presents as an ovoid, irreducible, painless swelling of variable size. It is very common in the perinatal period, and is produced by dilatation of the lower end of an incompletely closed processus vaginalis. Natural closure of the processus vaginalis is common in the first year of life. If the hydrocele persists surgical intervention may be advisable.

Encysted hydrocele of the (spermatic) cord is less common. It presents as a cystic swelling above the testis. It causes no trouble, but can be removed surgically.

Secondary hydrocele is not seen in childhood, but hydrocele may occur as a complication of mumps.

Varicocele

The definition of varicocele is difficult – in essence it is a varicose proliferation of the veins of the pampiniform plexus exceeding the 'norm'. Definition of the 'norm' is impossible. The left side is almost invariably affected. Right-sided varicocele only occurs in the very rare cases of situs inversus totalis. Varicocele occasionally leads to diminution in size of the homolateral testis, and may debar the candidate from service in the armed forces.

The only effective treatment is surgical, but this should not be lightly undertaken, as testicular atrophy may follow.

References

1. Scadding, J. G. (1977). Definition and clinical categories of asthma. In Clark, T. J. H. and Godfrey, S. (eds.) *Asthma*. p. 5. (London: Chapman and Hall)
2. Marks, B. E. and Hillier, V. F. (1983). General practitioners' views on asthma in childhood. *Br. Med. J.,* 287, 949
3. Meadow, S. R. (1977). How to use buzzer alarms to cure bed wetting. *Br. Med. J.,* 2, 1073
4. Sparks, J. P. (1978). The incidence of migraine in schoolchildren. A survey by the Medical Officers of Schools Association. *Practitioner,* 221, 407
5. Bille, B. (1962). Migraine in schoolchildren. *Acta Paediatr.,* 51 (suppl. 136), 13
6. David, T. J., Parris, M. R., Poynor, M., Hawnaur, T., Simm, S., Rigg, E. and McCrae, F. (1983). Reasons for late detection of hip dislocation in childhood. *Lancet,* 2, 147
7. Scorer, C. G. (1956). The incidence of incomplete descent of the testicle at birth. *Arch. Dis. Child.* 31, 198

CHAPTER 6

CHILDREN WITH SPECIAL EDUCATIONAL NEEDS

Introduction

It is not easy in a handbook such as this to summarize those medical conditions which will handicap a child during the course of his education.

The report of the Warnock Committee[1] makes it clear that many children experience problems of learning at some time during their school life, a far larger number than those with serious and overt handicaps. It estimates that up to one child in five is likely to require some form of special educational provision at some point in his school career. For all these children it is essential to check their neurological and developmental progress, and in particular those aspects which may affect their cognitive development. These include vision and hearing together with auditory and visual memory and recall. The Warnock report made it clear that the 'categories of handicap' defined in the Education Act 1944 are no longer acceptable or applicable. This was confirmed by the Education Act 1981 which brought into being a more detailed assessment procedure, involving a much wider team of professionals than before and much greater parental involvement in the choice of the type of education to be provided for a child with any handicap.

Educational provision for children with handicaps

The Education Act 1981 clearly states that it is the responsibility of the Health Authority to draw to the attention of the Local Education Authority any child who by reason of a medical condition will need special educational help. It remains the responsibility of the Education Authority to provide such help for all children of statutory school age, for children from the age of 2 years whose parents request it, and from birth for those profoundly handicapped by congenital conditions.

Although there is a medical component, this is largely advisory as the new procedures of assessment and recommendation are educationally orientated, but the need for close consultation between all the professionals concerned (teachers, doctors, nurses, educational psychologists, speech therapists, social workers, etc.) together with the parents is stressed. Annual reappraisal for all, and regular reassessment for the severely handicapped, are also requirements of the Act.

Integration into ordinary school is to be considered more widely, if necessary with special medical support services within the school. However, it is evident that there are children whose conditions render them so severely handicapped as to make this impossible. This includes the blind, the profoundly deaf, the severely emotionally disturbed and those with multiple handicaps such as physical disability combined with severe mental retardation. For these children special educational methods are provided in special classes or units within ordinary schools, or in separate special schools (which may be day or boarding) where treatment is part of the curriculum. Nursing and medical staff, such as physiotherapists and psychotherapists, are members of the school team.

All handicapped school leavers need special counselling and advice, which should be given at the most appropriate time for planning subject choices for examinations or vocational training. This is usually about 13 or 14 years, when the school doctor, teacher and careers adviser need to discuss the future with parents and pupil in terms of further and higher education or appropriate employment. For the severely handicapped the Departments of Employment and Social Services provide assessment, individual rehabilitation and vocational guidance.

Gifted children

School doctors should be aware that highly intelligent children may present behaviour problems, particularly when their high intelligence is not recognized due to underachievement. Even when recognized, the gifted child may require sensitive handling. The National Association for Gifted Children was founded in 1966 to foster the recognition of the peculiar needs of gifted children. The Association's leaflet describes some of the needs thus:

'A minority of gifted children – particularly those who fall into the unidentified group – may run into trouble of various kinds; they can be desperately lonely because their interests do not match with those of their peers; they can be regarded as "awkward customers" because of their unconventional behaviour in class and questioning attitude; they can become disturbed through frustration and boredom, or through imbalance between their intellectual and their emotional development; they can deliberately underachieve so as to be accepted by their classmates and teachers; they may even become delinquent'.

Only in the case of children with exceptional gifts for music and ballet is segregated schooling recommended. Doctors need to be alert to the possibility of disturbed behaviour being due to unrecognized high intelligence, and should call on the help of an educational psychologist if in doubt.

Further reading

A bibliography is available from the National Association fo Gifted Children, 1 South Audley Street, London W1Y 5DQ (Telephone: 01-499 1188).

Dyslexic children

It is of some interest that dyslexia as a handicap of healthy childrer was first described in 1896 by James Kerr[2], later to become Chiel School Medical Officer to the LCC and President of MOSA. He drew attention to the existence of mentally able children with 'bizarre defects' which led to grave difficulties in reading and spelling. He also recognized that 'slight cases are also met'. Interest in dyslexia waxed and waned until the late 1960s, when the disadvantage of dyslexic children in competing in public examinations led to the formation of dyslexia associations to press for greater understanding and reforms in the examination system. Until now, only the more bizarre and severe examples of dyslexia had been given much attention, and much of the published work on the subject was written by neurologists[3]. The development of screening tests, such as the Aston Index[4], which could be administered by lay people led to the discovery that learning difficulties were common, and comprised a spectrum of disability, which may involve predominantly auditory short-term memory, visual short-term memory or both, with or without confusion of laterality. Many children have minor degrees of weakness in these areas, and no two children are exactly the same. It is sometimes suggested empirically that a child subjected to the usual process of education whose reading age is 2 or more years below the mental age can be regarded as dyslexic. This ratio obviously has different implications according to the age of the child and presupposes accurate knowledge of the mental age, or IQ.

These matters are in the field of the educational psychologist rather than the doctor, and in 1979 the British Medical Association was asked to clarify the medical attitude to dyslexia. Its Board of Science concluded that dyslexia was not basically a medical problem, and issued the following statement:

'Dyslexia is essentially a learning disability which initially shows itself by difficulty in writing as opposed to speaking words. It tends to lessen as the child grows older, and is capable of considerable improvement especially when appropriate help is offered at the earliest opportunity. It is not due to intellectual inadequacy, or faulty teaching, nor is it associated with emotion or anatomical defects.

Quite frequently it is the family doctor or even a paediatrician to whom a child is brought with reading difficulties and such a child needs to be fully assessed both medically and psychologically. Certification of the disability, however, should be the responsibility of an educational psychologist, who should tell those concerned with the child's education what he or she could not do. Most doctors are not competent or willing to diagnose dyslexia without the assessment of an educational psychologist, and most dyslexic patients will be identified in the educational environment anyway, and hopefully be referred to an educational psychologist direct.

We very much hope that this is something which will be universally recognized by teachers as essentially a problem which does not need to concern doctors, and we have an understanding that the Schools Council will send the agreed report to all Local Education Authorities.

There is considerable variation in the availability of educational psychologists up and down the country, but we understand that every Educational Authority does have access to this service. There is also considerable variation in the way in which examination boards make allowances for children with dyslexia, and we have recommended that examination boards should be notified by head teachers well in advance of examination dates and be given a clear statement of the degree of disability in the individual – emphasizing that a medical certificate is not appropriate.

We very much hope that teachers will accept that this is something best recognized by them, and that they will refer to the specialists within their own authorities without necessarily referring to the family doctor, but it is important for doctors to know that this is the BMA recommendation, so that they may appropriately refer if such children are nevertheless brought to them by worried parents'.

School doctors are still likely to become involved in advising children, parents and schools in some cases of learning difficulty. They can be helpful in facilitating referral to an appropriate educational psychologist and in fostering good relations between the psychologist, the parents, the child and the teachers – both remedial teachers, if they are to be involved, and the classroom teachers, whose real difficulties in coping with dyslexic children in the classroom are not always appreciated. Although 'medical certificates' of dyslexia have been accepted by examining boards in the past, this is no longer the case, and the doctor should not attempt to provide one. The only reports which are now appropriate are from educational psychologists.

References

1. Cmnd 7212 (1978). *Special Educational Needs*. Report of the Committee of Enquiry into the Educational Needs of Handicapped Children. (London: HMSO)
2. Kerr, J. (1897). School hygiene in its mental, moral and physical aspects. Howard Medal Prize Essay. *J. R. Statist. Soc.*, 60, 613
3. Critchley, M. (1970). *The Dyslexic Child*. (London: William Heinemann Medical Books)
4. Newton, M. and Ratcliff, C. (1974). *The Aston Index*. (Birmingham: Aston University, and Wisbech: Learning Development Aids).

CHAPTER 7

SPORTS INJURIES AT SCHOOL

Introduction

Sport has played a very important part in school life in the independent sector for well over a century, and MOSA has concerned itself with sports injuries since its foundation in 1884. Since then there has been an enormous boom in participation in sport among schoolchildren and adults alike, and games are no longer the exclusive preoccupation of a boarding school elite. As a result, there has been a widening of interest in sports medicine to a point where some would regard it as a speciality in its own right. Certainly there are now many textbooks on sports injuries and sports medicine, and this Handbook cannot attempt to cover the same ground. Instead, this chapter aims to provide a concise overview for medical and non-medical staff, concentrating on the injuries which may be met with in school sports, and detailing practical points in their prevention and management.

Incidence

Weightman and Browne[1], who commented on the paucity of data on the incidence of sports injuries, were among the first to try to remedy the situation, apart from school doctors who have used their special opportunities to observe and record injuries in schools. Sparks[2] reviewed these in 1981, including his own unique records of 30 years at Rugby School: some details of these are presented in Appendix G (pp. 213–216). All series agree in showing that Rugby's own code of football causes more injuries than all other team games together: in the case of Rugby School nearly 200 per 10 000 player hours, with the head and neck being most frequently injured, followed by the ankle, hand and knee. Sparks summarized the implications of his observations as follows:

'All team games carry a quantifiable risk of injury. Rugby football is a game of physical contact, much of it violent. The injury rate for Rugby football is the highest of all games at this school. Even so, the more than 4500 boarders who have passed through the school in the past 30 years have each sustained, on average, only two football injuries, and few have been serious'.

The type of injury which has caused most concern recently is injury to the cervical cord, leading as it may to death or permanent tetraplegia. It occurs most commonly as a consequence of accidents in horse riding, motor cycling, trampolining and diving, but until the 1970s was regarded as a rarity in team sports. It is now clear, however, that its incidence in Rugby football has greatly increased. Data are still sketchy, but a retrospective survey[3] of injury to English schoolboys found 12 cases causing death or permanent tetraplegia in the 6 years from 1973 to 1978, all due to Rugby football. A survey[4] in New Zealand covering the same period found 54 cases of injury, five of which were fatal, with a quarter of the players being under 17 at the time of the accident. Attempts are now being made to set up a reliable register of injuries.

Prevention

For any sport adequate training and skilled coaching reduce the number of injuries in that particular activity; it should never be a hurried beginning-of-term affair. Weight and circuit training and the teaching of skills all play an important part, but adequate warming up before every game and sporting activity is essential: without it the risk of soft tissue injury is greatly increased.

Locomotor fitness includes muscle strength and endurance, flexibility and other skeletal adaptations, some of which may be specific to particular sports. Before competition is undertaken it is essential that locomotor fitness is produced by carefully graduated training. Cardiovascular-respiratory fitness, involving mainly oxygen uptake and supply to working muscles, is most relevant in sports events in which physical endurance is important.

Various methods of fitness training are commonly used.

Circuit training

A sequence of exercises is performed as fast as possible *en route* around the gymnasium. The number of repetitions and the nature of each exercise vary according to the subject's age, physique and degree of fitness. The total time taken for the circuit is timed, usually by the individual, with a large training clock. Circuit training is in use by coaches for a wide variety of different sports and is an excellent method of producing both locomotor and cardiovascular-respiratory types of fitness. It can also incorporate skills of certain sports, although general circuits can be tailored to subjects of any age who are wanting to improve their overall fitness.

Weight training

Strength may be developed by exercising to exhaustion using heavy weights for a small number of repetitions. Local muscle endurance is produced by the use of lighter weights with a large number of repetitions. Springs, pulleys and a variety of exercisers, or body-weight (of the subject or that of a partner) may be used instead of weights. Specific muscle groups may be strengthened to counteract weaknesses which are detracting from performance.

Weight training in schools should be carefully supervised to avoid muscle strains, particularly of the back. Some adolescents are enthusiasts for weight training for its own sake, and may need to be restrained. There is a tendency for some sportsmen to try to prove their strength and virility by using heavy weights, and this negates the purpose of training. It needs to be remembered that some exercises provided by weight training equipment are inappropriate for post-injury rehabilitation: for example isotonic quadriceps exercises are not suitable for knee injuries, which require repeated straight leg raising with a weighted boot.

Interval training

This consists of a number of fast laps with regular controlled intervals of rest between each lap. It is used mainly by swimmers and runners and produces especially cardiovascular-respiratory fitness. It can be varied to apply to differing events and sports, and produces maximum fitness when the resting intervals are timed to finish when the heart rate falls to 120 per minute. With the aid of a training clock it is possible for the subject to vary the resting intervals according to when this heart rate is reached.

Flexibility training

Exercises to increase joint mobility and the extensibility of muscles and tendons are especially important in early season training and when heavy weight training has been undertaken. Flexibility training should be incorporated into a warm-up routine to be performed before every game and practice.

Skills training

This may vary from practices designed to enhance the specialist skills of particular sports to practice matches, time trials or other procedures.

The governing bodies of most sports produce coaching manuals containing fitness training appropriate to their particular sport. Some fitness training is specific to the sport concerned. Instances such as that of the outstanding test match fast bowler playing social Sunday afternoon tennis and producing tendinitis of his bowling shoulder are well known. Similarly the international oarsman who competes in an unusually long club event and sustains tenosynovitis in both wrists illustrates that fitness may be event-specific within individual sports.

If lack of exercise is a risk factor for cardiovascular disease in adults it is likely that sport contributes significantly to the maintenance of health and fitness during later life. It is important for schools to encourage the individual and team games which may be enjoyed into adult life. Many schoolchildren do not excel at or enjoy the major team sports, so the provision of a wide variety of games options is important. In addition to the traditional sports, others should be provided such as archery, fencing, judo, swimming activities (such as life-saving, synchronized swimming and survival swimming) together with modern educational gymnastics (or movement training) and modern educational dance.

The skilful and enthusiastic coach may motivate schoolchildren to intense effort both in training and competition. It is therefore important to be certain that children are basically healthy before severe training is undertaken. It must be remembered that some apparently trivial virus infections may cause undetected myocarditis, and there have been occasional instances of sudden death from this cause on the sports field. It is therefore a wise practice for school doctors to forbid pupils all forms of physical exercise for at least a week after an attack of influenza and similar illnesses.

Head injuries

Minor head injury due to sport is very common, but serious injury is rare. In a review of 84 000 patients with head injuries attending accident and emergency departments in Scotland in 1974, Lindsay *et al.*[5] found that only 0.3% had sports injuries requiring admission and only 2.7% of all admissions for head injury were sustained during athletic or competitive recreational activities. Briscoe[6], on the other hand, noted a steady increase in minor head injuries in Eton College, and attributed this to the rising popularity of Rugby football, more aggressive play, and a greater awareness by the school staff of the need for medical attention of pupils with symptoms and signs of minor head injury. Additional factors were the introduction of a concrete swimming pool and of new sports such as judo. Thus, approximately 1% of boys at Eton suffer a minor head injury each year, compared with 4% at Rugby where Rugby football is the principal game in the Advent Term.

In the Scottish study the commonest cause of head injury requiring hospital admission in schoolchildren was golf, but in only one of these was the injury caused by the ball; 13 out of 14 were caused by the club. The authors point out that these figures reflect the popularity of the game in Scotland. The next most common cause was horse riding. By far the commonest cause of fatal head injury from sport in Scotland was climbing.

Minor head injury is defined as head injury without fracture, prolonged unconsciousness or neurological sequelae. This is synonymous with concussion when there has been loss of consciousness, however brief, or a period of amnesia. If the patient cannot remember the blow on the head, he can be considered as concussed. Regrograde amnesia is loss of memory for a period preceding injury, and is usually brief, but its duration gives some indication of the severity of the injury. Post-traumatic amnesia is the period of loss of memory after the injury. Briscoe[6] recognizes a condition of subconcussion in which consciousness is not lost but clinical and experimental evidence suggests that there is nevertheless some nerve cell damage. Headache is experienced by only about half of all patients with minor head injury. In a minority, there is also nausea or vomiting, dizziness, disorientation and temporarily blurred or double vision. Increase in intensity of headache, repeated vomiting and a deteriorating level of consciousness are serious signs which should alert the attendant to the possibility of a rise in intracranial pressure due to bleeding.

Prevention

In sports with a high risk of head injury, such as horse riding and climbing, protective head gear must be worn. In contact sports, mouth guards reduce the risk of concussion by diminishing the force transmitted through the temporomandibular joint from blows on the face. This is secondary to their main purpose of preventing dental injuries, and they are therefore dealt with in the section on dental injury on p. 108.

Management

The possibly fatal consequences of serious head injury combined with the frequent occurrence of minor injuries present some difficulties in deciding on a policy of management, but it is important that every school should formulate such a policy and make sure it is widely understood. The doctor must bear in mind that if his policy is unrealistically restrictive it may be more honoured in the breach than the observance, and therefore counterproductive.

In serious injuries associated with coma, there is a risk of airway obstruction, and first aid measures may be necessary to ensure the patency of the airway and prevent inhalation of vomit. The most feared complication of head injury is the extradural or subdural haematoma developing after an apparently trivial injury and a lucid interval, and, rare though this is, it colours the management of every head injury. Finally, and perhaps most difficult of all, is the risk of cumulative damage from repeated injuries. Some sports, such as boxing, have a mandatory policy of restriction after head injury, but this is not the case in contact sports played at school. There is no precise unanimity in the matter, but what follows is considered to be a reasonable policy to follow in schools.

If a player falls after a knock on the head but is instantly on his feet again he can safely continue playing.

If he falls and is unable to get to his feet for 10 seconds, and is then somewhat confused, he must go off the field and remain off for the rest of the game. It is the referee's responsibility to enforce this, and the player must be sent to the sanatorium where he should be admitted for observation for 24 hours. If there is no sanatorium, he should attend the nearest hospital Accident and Emergency department. The question of whether to arrange skull X-rays is controversial. In view of the large number of minor head injuries from sport and the very small number of fractures[6], most school doctors are content to rely on clinical judgement. Lindsay *et al.*[5]

recommend X-rays if there is post-traumatic amnesia and depression of level of consciousness, with admission to hospital of all patients with a fracture, however well they may seem, because of the increased risk of haematoma. After an injury requiring sanatorium admission the player should not resume contact sport for at least a week, and then only with the permission of the doctor.

If a player is unconscious for over a minute, with complete amnesia for half an hour or more, the position is more serious. In these circumstances a steeplechase jockey is not allowed to ride again for 3 weeks, and then only after being cleared to do so by a specialist with experience in head injuries. It would be prudent to subject school sportsmen to at least as rigorous a restriction.

There remains the problem of the player who has more than one episode of unconsciousness. This requires careful attention because the expectation of the player and his coach of early return after an apparently minor injury contrasts with medical knowledge that repeated injuries have a cumulative effect[7] even if they do not reach the severity of traumatic encephalopathy seen in boxers and jockeys. After a second head injury causing unconsciousness in one season, it is wise to keep the player off contact sport for a minimum of 4 weeks. With repeated episodes even more caution is necessary, and it is very occasionally necessary to advise a player who has had several episodes of unconsciousness with post-traumatic amnesia to give up contact sport for good. Similar care must be exercised if a player shows signs of the postconcussion syndrome, with persistent headaches, dizziness, irritability and poor concentration.

Neck injuries

Neck injuries are among the most serious which can affect schoolchildren as a result of sport. Fracture-dislocation of the cervical spine, according to the level at which it occurs and the degree of damage to the spinal cord, causes death or paralysis below the level of the lesion – paralysis which may recover partially or completely, or may leave the patient a lifelong tetraplegic. There is good reason to believe that the adolescent skeleton is more vulnerable to stress that that of the young adult. The mechanism of injury is forced flexion or extension of the neck combined with rotation. It can occur as a result of a fall on the head, commonly from a horse or diving board; from loss of control when trampolining; or from Rugby football. The increase in neck injuries from Rugby football seems to date from the early 1970s, and must be related not only to the increasing popularity of the sport but also to changes in the way it is played. Scher[8] was the first to draw attention to the enormous forces applied to the neck of front row forwards in the set scrum, and scrum collapses have caused a proportion of these injuries. However, serious injuries also occur in the tackle, ruck and loose play.

Prevention

Strict care needs to be exercised in the control of diving and gymnastics.

The prevention of neck injuries from Rugby football is one of the greatest challenges faced by the Rugby Football Unions, who have devoted a great deal of skilled attention to it. Laws have been changed with a view to preventing injury in the set scrum and the ruck, and advice given on coaching for skilled tackling and safe play in general. Players are advised to carry out preseason exercises specifically designed to strengthen the muscles of the neck and shoulder girdle, and referees are instructed in the firm control of the game. In schools it is imperative that the closest attention be given to all these matters, and above all players must not be inappropriately matched for size, skill and experience. Boys with long, slender necks are particularly vulnerable in the front row of the scrum. MOSA has for many years urged that junior teams should be selected by weight rather than by chronological age, the reasons for which are explained in Chapter 4 (p. 52). A particularly heavy onus falls on those who arrange matches between school teams and old boys' sides to see that immature players are not pitched against strong adults, particularly in the scrum. Schoolboys should only play with adult clubs in exceptional circumstances, and the doctor's advice should be sought before they do so.

The occurrence of tetraplegia in schoolboys has led to the appreciation of a distressing lack of insurance cover, in contrast to other countries. It is strongly advised that schoolboy Rugby players should be adequately insured, a matter that is dealt with on p. 113.

Management

Although the degree of permanent damage may be determined at the moment of injury, correct first aid treatment is essential to prevent any further damage to the spinal cord. If the casualty complains of sensations of electric shock, tingling or numbness he should be moved on a stretcher. If there is paralysis, the ambulance (or helicopter, if available) should be brought on to the field of play, in the case of a Rugby injury. The player may fall in the prone position, and a BBC film, available to Rugby clubs, shows how the casualty should be turned into the supine position. It is debatable whether this should be attempted, as any mistake by those turning the player can have catastrophic results.

Cervical splints which can easily be applied on the field in order to immobilize the cervical spine are now available. These make the handling of neck casualties easier and safer and it is strongly recommended that every Rugby-playing school should have a splint and ensure that it is kept with standard first aid equipment so that it is always available if needed.

Eye injuries

Court games are responsible for most injuries to the eyeball, due to the high velocity and small diameter of the ball. Squash causes the majority of serious sports injuries to the eye. The shuttlecock in badminton may have a similar effect. Apart from corneal abrasions, the commonest injuries involve the anterior chamber (hyphaema) or retina. In either case there will be sudden blurring of vision, which should always mean immediate referral to a doctor.

Black eye, or orbital haematoma, frequently occurs in contact sports, but damage to the eye itself is uncommon. The doctor must be on his guard if there is double vision or enophthalmos, because these may indicate a 'blow-out' fracture of the orbital floor.

Finally, the high myope is at special risk of traumatic detachment of the retina.

Prevention

Those who wear spectacles should always have plastic lenses for small ball games. They should not wear spectacles for Association or Rugby football, but contact lenses are safe. As there is a considerable toll of serious eye injuries in squash, there has been strong pressure in some quarters for eye protection, such as wrap-around frames with polycarbonate lenses, or padded visors. Unfortunately this advice has not met with general acceptance among players or with the Squash Racquets Association.

Short-sighted people should not box, as the risk of traumatic detachment of the retina in myopes is well recognized by the boxing authorities. It is not so well appreciated by Rugby players and coaches. People with severe myopia would be well advised not to play the more traumatic contact sports because of this risk, and should receive the support of their school doctor in excusing them these sports.

Management

Cases of hyphaema or suspected retinal damage are best referred to a hospital eye department for assessment and treatment. Hyphaema resolves with bed rest, but there is a risk of secondary haemorrhage some days later, and this may cause permanent visual impairment.

If a 'blow-out' fracture is suspected the patient must be referred for X-ray, and, if a fracture is confirmed, to a faciomaxillary or ophthalmic surgeon. Treatment is usually expectant.

Dental injuries

Fractures of the incisors are remarkably common in school age children, and are frequently caused by sport. Sparks[2] recorded 157 cases of fractured teeth (3 per 10 000 player hours) in his 30-year survey of Rugby injuries (see Appendix G). A fractured tooth usually means that dental treatment will be needed at intervals throughout the patient's life. A blow on the face sometimes knocks out an incisor from the root without fracturing it.

Prevention

Fractures of the teeth can largely be prevented by mouth guards if they are properly fitted[9]. This is best done by a dental surgeon, but it is not available at National Health Service expense. The cost could well be regarded as a reasonable insurance premium against the life-long discomfort and expense which may result from a dental fracture. Opinions differ about the value of cheaper mouthguards fitted by a nurse or lay person, but it is certain that appliances bought over the counter are not satisfactory.

Mouthguards are recommended for all serious Rugby and hockey players who are well enough motivated to wear them. This applies to younger as well as older players, though new guards will have to be fitted as the face grows.

Management

All those concerned with contact sports should understand that if an incisor is knocked out completely it may well survive if promptly replaced in the socket. The tooth should therefore be found and brought at once with the patient to the dentist, doctor or nurse; if none is available it is not difficult for a lay person to replace the tooth. If very dirty it can be washed in warm saline; otherwise it is best kept warm and moist in the patient's mouth. It can then be easily reinserted in the socket and kept in place by gentle pressure. Tetanus prophylaxis should be given if the patient has not had an injection of tetanus vaccine in the past 5 years. The patient should be seen by a dentist as soon as possible after replacement of the tooth. The outlook is usually good if it is done within 20 minutes of the injury.

Patients with fractured teeth should be seen as soon as possible by a dentist, particularly if the pulp is seen to have been exposed by the fracture.

Fractures and dislocations

Fractures of the long bones, clavicle, ribs, metacarpals, metatarsals and phalanges all occur commonly in sport, and if a fracture is suspected the patient must be referred to hospital for X-ray and treatment. Generally speaking the outlook for all these fractures in adolescents is very good, but certain diagnostic and therapeutic pitfalls are worth mentioning.

Fractures of the carpal scaphoid, notoriously prone to complications in adults, seldom give lasting trouble in the adolescent so long as the diagnosis is made on radiological and clinical grounds, and an appropriate plaster applied.

Mallet deformities of the fingers occur most commonly in Rugby football and basketball. In contrast to such cases in the adult, where the results are very poor, immobilization for 6 weeks in a mallet splint usually ensures a cure irrespective of whether the injury is one of tendon alone or tendon plus bony fragment. Injury to the flexor tendons can also occur: hand injuries must be examined carefully to ensure early diagnosis and treatment.

Stress fractures of the tibia, lower end of the fibula, and metatarsals are most commonly seen in cross country runners and gymnasts. The diagnosis can easily be missed. Stress fracture of the upper third of the fibula is seen in hurdlers.

Dislocations, except for those of the patella, occur most commonly in Rugby football. Reduction of the early case is usually easy either without analgesia or under intravenous diazepam or pethidine. Recurrent dislocation of the shoulder can cause great inconvenience to the games player, and usually requires surgery.

The knee and ankle

The knee is commonly injured in all types of sport. After an acute injury there is usually an effusion which may make a precise diagnosis impossible. Moderate, lax effusions can be treated expectantly with intensive quadriceps exercises and a knee support, but haemarthroses and tense effusions need prompt aspiration. Referral to an orthopaedic surgeon experienced in arthroscopy should not be delayed, as early treatment has greatly improved the prognosis in knee injury.

In ankle injuries the most important complication is the loss of proprioceptive control which can lead to long-term problems. Early physiotherapy is therefore important to rehabilitate the ankle joint.

Osteochondritis and overuse injury

Many conditions of adolescent sportsmen are related in part to overuse, this is to say, to a degree of stress on the developing skeletal system sufficient to cause symptoms. It is now believed that most types of osteochondritis come into this category. This was recognized by a distinguished school doctor in the early years of MOSA. Farquharson[10] described a strain of the quadriceps tendon at its insertion to the tibial tubercle which many years later received the misleading name of Osgood–Schlatter's disease, setting a fashion for eponyms in a series of related conditions which are in no sense diseases.

Osgood–Schlatter's disease, which is very familiar to all school doctors, is probably a traumatic apophysitis of the tibial tubercle and causes no long-term disability. It commonly occurs around the years of puberty and is exacerbated by kneeling. Pain is the only indication for restriction of activity, and some patients have to avoid heavy ball games for some months. This is particularly frustrating as the condition usually occurs in the most energetic footballers. Specific treatment, such as immobilization in a plaster cylinder, is very seldom necessary or desirable. The place of local steroid injections is controversial.

Apophysitis also occurs in the calcaneum, causing painful heels which characteristically occur early in the football season when playing surfaces are often hard. Rest from all exercise for a period may be necessary, followed by cushioning of the heel with a sorbo-rubber insole. Running on hard surfaces should be avoided as far as possible.

Osteochondritis dissecans is a condition of avascular necrosis of the articular surface of a femoral condyle, sometimes leading to a loose body in the joint. This, too, is usually seen in the most active adolescents, and referral to an orthopaedic surgeon is necessary for its management.

Osteochondritis of the spine is common in adolescence and is often symptomless. In some it causes chronic backache for several months, but it is self-limiting, and sport is not contraindicated.

Chondromalacia patellae is a particularly frustrating cause of chronic knee pain, especially in adolescent girls. There is retropatellar inflammation and roughening which may lead to crepitus and an effusion. Treatment is singularly ineffective. The schoolgirl or boy with this condition, which is sometimes known as 'painful patella syndrome', should be advised to do regular quadriceps exercises and restrict athletic activities to those which do not seriously aggravate the pain. Referral to an orthopaedic surgeon is desirable for severe cases.

The high performance training required for young gymnasts and some athletes subjects the body to considerable stress. As yet there is no definite evidence of what harm this does, but concern has been expressed in many quarters. The school doctor may sometimes be in a position to discourage the excessive ambitions of parents and coaches when he believes the young person is at risk, particularly when an overuse injury has been diagnosed.

Prevention

Overuse injuries cannot be totally prevented, but their toll could certainly be reduced by a sensible attitude to training, skill in coaching and care over equipment. This particularly applies to footwear, as some of the stresses applied to athletes' lower limbs and hips can be mitigated by modern well-designed running shoes.

Soft tissue injuries

The majority of sports injuries come into the category of soft tissue injuries. Despite the susceptibility of coaches to marketing exploitation of impressive-looking applications and dressings, the time-worn methods have not become any less effective. The mnemonic ICE, standing for ice, compression and elevation, remains the most effective first aid treatment for virtually all sprains, strains and contusions. It is important that ice is not applied direct or for too long, as cold injury can result. An application of melting ice in a cloth at 4°C for 5 minutes is sufficient. After injury, physiotherapy is often helpful for rehabilitation. The use of non-steroidal anti-inflammatory agents is becoming popular, but there is as yet no good evidence of their efficacy.

Lacerations

Lacerations can occur accidentally in all sport, football boot studs and running shoe spikes being among the commoner causes.

Prevention

It should be possible to prevent most lacerations by careful attention to safety procedures, care with running spikes and, above all, unceasing attention to the state of studs in football boots. This is a responsibility of players, coaches and referees alike.

Management

The school doctor who is skilled in suturing can prevent many long hours of waiting in busy Accident and Emergency departments. He will be careful to exclude underlying injury, carry out proper debridement and ensure a good cosmetic result, as well as checking on tetanus prevention (see p. 39). Many lacerations which would formerly have been sutured can now be closed satisfactorily with sterile skin closure strips. In international sport there is a growing tendency for players to resume play immediately after suturing. The school doctor should exercise more caution, and will usually want to exclude the player from further activity until sound healing has taken place.

Insurance

Every year a small number of schoolchildren are permanently disabled by a sports injury. While injuries due to negligence or road traffic accidents are generously compensated through the courts, and many adult sports carry mandatory insurance cover, the schoolchild accidentally injured in the course of a game at school will receive no compensation unless insurance cover has been arranged. It is not sufficient to expect parents to take the initiative for individual accident insurance, and it is now recognized, at least in independent schools, that insurance against accidental injury is a responsibility which must be accepted by the school, irrespective of who finally pays the premium. A number of schemes have been drawn up by insurance companies, and school authorities are very strongly advised to participate. The best policies cover all sport and adventure activity officially organized by the school, and require registration of every pupil in the scheme. Death benefit is limited by law to £1000 in the case of a minor, but the most important provision is for adequate cover for the lifelong costs of permanent total disablement: £100 000 should be regarded as a minimum, and some schemes now insure for £200 000. The premiums for group schemes are much lower than for individual accident policies. Details can be obtained from the Hon. Secretary of MOSA and from the Independent Schools Joint Council.

References

1. Weightman, D. and Browne, R. C. (1974). Injuries in association and rugby football. *Br. J. Sports Med.*, 8, 183
2. Sparks, J. P. (1981). Half a million hours of Rugby Football. *Br. J. Sports Med.*, 15, 30
3. Hoskins, T. (1979). Rugby injuries to the cervical spine in English schoolboys. *Practitioner*, 223, 365
4. Burry, H. C. and Gowland, H. (1979). Cervical injury in Rugby football – a New Zealand survey. *Br. J. Sports Med.*, 15, 56
5. Lindsay, K. W., McLatchie, G. and Jennett, B. (1980). Serious head injury in sport. *Br. Med. J.*, 281, 789
6. Briscoe, J. H. D. (1978). Minor head injury in adolescent boys. *Practitioner*, 221, 751
7. Gronwall, D. and Wrightson, P. (1975). Cumulative effect of concussion. *Lancet* 2, 995
8. Scher, A. T. (1977). Rugby injuries to the cervical spinal cord. *South Afr. Med. J.*, 51, 473
9. Turner, C. H., (1977). Mouth protectors. *Br. Dent. J.*, 143, 82
10. Farquharson, R. (1885). *School Hygiene and Diseases Incidental to School Life*. (London: Smith, Elder)

CHAPTER 8

SAFETY AT SCHOOL

Introduction

Sports injuries and their prevention have been dealt with in Chapter 7. Schools are subject to the Health and Safety at Work Act 1974, and safety at school covers a wide field. The Department of Education and Science publishes a series of booklets[1-5] which it recommends should be available in all schools. This chapter will not attempt to duplicate the advice given in these important booklets. Most topics not already mentioned will be noted briefly, but swimming pool safety and adventure training merit fuller treatment.

The Health and Safety at Work Act 1974

The purpose of the Act and consequent regulations is to promote and encourage high standards of health and safety at work, and schools are included in the places of work to which the Act applies. It is a statutory requirement for employers to publish a written safety policy and appoint a safety officer.

The Notification of Accidents and Dangerous Occurrences Regulations 1980 require that accidents resulting in death or major injury to a pupil (including major sports injuries during games taking place on premises controlled by the school) should be reported to the Health and Safety Executive. The responsibility for notification lies with the local education authorities for maintained schools and the governing bodies for independent schools. School doctors should therefore report such accidents and injuries to their safety officer. Major injury is defined as:

(a)　fracture of the skull, spine or pelvis;

(b)　fracture of any bone
　　　(i)　in the arm, other than a bone in the wrist or hand,
　　　(ii)　in the leg, other than a bone in the ankle or foot;

(c)　amputation of a hand or foot;

(d)　the loss of sight of an eye;

(e)　any other injury which results in the person being admitted
　　　into hospital as an inpatient for more than 24 hours, unless
　　　that person is detained only for observation.

Leaflets giving further details are available from the Health and Safety Executive, Room 158, Baynards House, 1 Chepstow Place, London W2 4TF (telephone: 01-229 3456, ext. 6586).

Swimming pool safety

Adequate supervision by a life-saver trained in the use of mouth-to-mouth artificial respiration is essential at all times because of the possibility of drowning, which may follow even trivial mishaps, as well as vasovagal attacks and fits. The preservation of good pool discipline also prevents other accidents such as skidding on slippery pool surrounds and collisions of swimmers. Pools should be strictly out of bounds after dances and parties at which alcohol has been consumed.

Diving accidents

In recent years, there has been a greater awareness of the risks of diving and very large sums have been awarded by the courts following spinal injuries from this cause. A code of practice has been agreed by a number of interested national organisations. Swimming should not be allowed near diving installations which are in use and there should be physical separation of swimmers and divers in these circumstances.

A table of minimum recommended depths of water is shown for various heights of firm diving boards. If spring boards are used, the depth of water should include an increment which is equal to the lift given by the springboard. The water depths are calculated on the assumption that the diving is supervised and that good order and discipline are maintained. Pupils should be instructed not to dive vertically into swimming pools except in an adequate deep end, and if public, parents or staff are allowed to use the pool, a notice should be prominently displayed saying 'No vertical diving'.

Recommended minimum water depths for diving for adults and adolescents

There should be no diving at all, not even racing dives, in less than 0.9 metres of water.

Bath side	2.5 metres
1 metre *firm* board	3.0 metres
2 metre *firm* board	3.5 metres
3 metre *firm* board	3.8 metres

For spring boards, add a depth of water equal to the height of the lift off the board.

For prepubertal children (for example at preparatory schools) subtract 0.5 metres from these depths.

Adventure training in schools

Adventure training now covers many differing activities as schools broaden the scope of their pupils' interests and capabilities. Certain factors of safety and health are common to all these activities and are discussed below. Problems related to individual activities will be referred to in later paragraphs.

Exposure (hypothermia)

The following instructions should be printed on a card (causes and symptoms on one side, treatment on the other).

Exposure (hypothermia) is a lowering of the internal body core temperature which will affect vital organs, such as the brain and heart. It can occur even in midsummer if the weather is bad.

Causes

Primary	Cold	a combination of two factors
	Wind	increases the danger
	Rain	

Secondary	Fatigue
	Anxiety or fear
	Thinness

Symptoms

Unreasonable behaviour
Lethargy, lack of response to orders, etc. ⎫ One of these
Persistent stumbling   ⎪ symptoms alone
Irrational outbursts of energy   ⎬ is enough to
Slurred speech   ⎪ act as a warning
Uncontrollable shivering   ⎭
Dimness of vision

Treatment

It is vital to stop further heat loss

(1) Stop and shelter immediately (buildings, tent or, at the very least, a windbreak).
(2) Blanket or sleeping bag – and polythene bag or 'space' blanket.
(3) Hot drinks and sugar by mouth.
(4) Mouth-to-mouth resuscitation may be needed.

DO NOT encourage patient to try to walk on (even after he has apparently recovered).
DO NOT try to warm him by
  giving alcohol by mouth,
  rubbing the skin,
  the use of hot water bottles.
Get motor transport as near to the patient as possible. A stretcher should only be used for a very short distance.

The card should be enclosed in a waterproof transparent cover, one carried by the leader and a second by his 'number two'. The instructions may appear to be rather peremptory, but in a howling gale or a rainstorm there is no time to read lengthy instructions with complicated physiological explanations written on a sodden rapidly disintegrating piece of paper.

If there is one case of exposure in the party, then the rest are probably dangerously near the same state. The leader himself will also probably be affected to some degree – this will make him less likely to notice the onset of symptoms in other members of the party, and appreciate the danger.

Prevention is better than the cure – always turn back or make for shelter in good time if the weather is worsening.

The traditional remedies – alcohol by mouth (even if it is brought by a St. Bernard dog!), rubbing the skin, hot water bottles – give the patient a feeling of warmth by raising the skin temperature. This rise, however, is produced by an increased blood flow through the skin, and this extra blood has to come from the body core. The end result is a lowering of the body core temperature – the very danger you are trying to prevent.

Heat exhaustion

On a hot day – in temperatures over 24°C (75°F) – the sweating brought on by physical exertion can cause heat exhaustion. This is due to the associated loss of sodium chloride (sweat contains 0.25% of sodium chloride).

The symptoms are giddiness and nausea followed by a typical 'faint' (cold, pale clammy skin, dilated pupils, and a rapid weak pulse; the temperature is subnormal, and the blood pressure low). Muscular cramps are often a premonitory symptom.

Prevention

The drinking water carried should have enough salt added to make it a 0.1% saline solution. This will replace the chloride loss.

Treatment

The treatment is rest, if possible in the shade out of the heat, and giving 0.1% saline solution by mouth.

Leadership

Whatever the activity, the leader must be known to be both competent technically and to possess the maturity to lead, control and encourage parties of young people. Personality and experience are most important. Although certificates in themselves should not be the main basis by which a teacher's capability to lead groups on dangerous activities is judged, if a teacher does attend a suitable course or reach a recognized level of competence, this enables a headmaster to assess the leader's ability to take a group to the Himalayas, say, rather than the Lake District.

Courses are available leading to the following leadership certificates:

Mountain walking and climbing

Mountain Walking Leader Certificates (Summer and Winter). Courses and assessment are run by the Mountain Walking Leader Training Scheme.

Canoeing

A graded test scheme is run by the British Canoe Union for both novice and expert.

Diving

The British Sub-Aqua Club runs a good system for divers and instructors at all levels of expertise.

Caving

Very good assessment and training courses are run in Yorkshire by the National Caving Association.

Sailing

The National Sailing Centre at Cowes operates a country-wide system of certification and courses.

Skiing

The British Association of Ski Instructors (BASI) organizes courses and assessment at different levels of skill.

Windsurfing

Training is offered by all recognized schools belonging to the Sailboard Association.

Planning

There is a fine line between the well-planned adventure which extends children towards their physical and mental limits and the event which pushes them beyond those limits, risking injury or death. Careful assessment of the risks is vital to good planning, drawing on experience or gathering information, particularly on climatic conditions. For example, what in summer will be a pleasant scramble to the summit of Snowdon will in winter become a major effort involving special equipment and requiring the capacity to deal with snow and ice conditions.

Fitness

Most accidents to school parties in the hills are caused by problems associated with fitness, both physical and mental. All leaders must be aware of the weak links in their parties and plan accordingly, since children can progress to exposure very rapidly when exhausted in wet, cold conditions. When this happens the fault lies with the leader, who must always assess the risks of this happening beforehand and turn back or bivouac in good time to avoid it.

There is growing awareness of the importance of preliminary fitness training within the club or school before going on the hills or water.

Clothing and equipment

Great improvements have been made in the clothing and equipment available for adventure activities. While this has made many activities safer, paradoxically it introduces new dangers if leaders rely on equipment at the expense of their own judgement. It is practice and experience coupled with these new improvements that can lead to the broadening of horizons.

Clothing for an expedition must be appropriate to the conditions expected and there is no standard issue which covers all imaginable trips. The following notes may help a leader to decide what is appropriate for his planned mountain trip.

Boots

Many of the new lightweight mountain boots lack the stiffness of sole and ankle support to be adequate all the year round. Lightweight leather boots are the answer for long distance low level walking and for summer fell walking. For winter use, pupils should be equipped with vibram-soled mountain boots which are reasonably stiff in the sole and provide good ankle support. Blisters can be a major problem and are prevented by ensuring well-fitting boots and allowing time for the feet to get used to them.

Socks

These should be either of the traditional woollen type or of the newer loopstitch, which forms a cushion between foot and boot and acts as a wick to remove sweat.

Trousers

These should be quick-drying, comfortable, warm and loose-fitting. Knee-length breeches are ideal provided very heavy materials are avoided. Tracksuit trousers and jeans should not be worn.

Shirts and sweaters

Shirts of wool or thick cotton such as football shirts are suitable. Fibrepile jackets and the traditional oiled wool sweaters provide good further insulation, the jackets having the advantage that the material is still insulating when wet and is virtually indestructible. They are not very windproof and normally need a windproof anorak as outer cover. Nylon shirts should never be worn.

Hats and gloves

Much body heat is lost through the head and wrists. The standard wool balaclava is an ideal and economic head cover and oiled wool mitts with an added waterproof outer are the standard gloves. Ski gloves are not suitable for British wet, cold conditions.

Outer cover

All groups must have good waterproof outer cover, both jacket and trousers. Thin nylon is not ideal for this purpose and neoprene is recommended. The jacket should ideally have a full zip and hood. The condensation problem has been eased by the development of special materials such as Goretex. These allow moisture to pass out without allowing water in, but are more expensive and are not recommended for heavy use by school groups.

Rucksacks

Both frame sacks and ergonomic sacks, which have partly replaced them, can be recommended. The latter are lighter and often more comfortable than earlier rucksacks. Young people should not normally carry more than 30 lb sacks unless on a major trip. All rucksacks leak to some extent so a plastic bag should be used to protect the contents.

With regard to clothing, it is important that the group leader should ensure that groups are maintaining the right clothing for the task in hand. Overdressed parties can lead to exhaustion just as easily as underdressed ones. Always check that group members have the correct kit before starting the trip.

Extra equipment

Personal

Spare sweater and shirt, map, compass, whistle, thermos flask or water bottle, rations for the day, torch if planning a winter walk.

Group kit

Each group of eight should have:

(a)   Two survival (polythene) bags or a group emergency shelter.

(b)   One sleeping bag (kept in a plastic bag).

(c)   Emergency rations plus small stove and fuel.

(d)   Two torches with spare batteries.

(e)   First aid kit containing dressings, plasters, aspirin, thermometer, scissors, bandages, antiseptic cream, etc.

(f)   A 50 ft length of rope if climbing is involved.

(g)   A miniflare pack for more serious expeditions (no gun licence required).

(h)   An extra warm garment, e.g. duvet jacket, carried by the leader for emergency use.

Canoeing equipment

All canoes must have adequate buoyancy and end-toggles; and must be well repaired with no jagged fibreglass edges. Spray decks if used should have a panic cord to help removal under water. There should be no odd ropes, loose laces or untied waist cords which could snag. Buoyancy aids are used by many canoeists in place of the less comfortable and bulkier life jackets, but for white water and surfing, helmets and wetsuits should be worn. There is a real risk of hypothermia on British rivers in winter and great attention should be paid to proper insulation. Wet, cold hands are not only painful but very dangerous: wetsuit neoprene gloves and insulation of alloy shafted paddles will help reduce heat loss from the hands. A vehicle to meet the canoeing group at various points down the river and allow warming up is highly desirable.

All canoeists should be aware of the risks associated with wet, cold conditions and be able to recognize the early signs of hypothermia. Since sudden immersion in cold water can lead to headaches and possible blackouts, leaders should always watch carefully and be prepared to assist a canoeist off the water if necessary. All canoe leaders should carry with them a safety line (throw bag), some repair tape and simple first aid kit.

Diving

All would-be divers who hope to progress to the use of aqualungs must be medically examined before they take their first open water dives. The British Sub-Aqua Club provides details of the examination required for school doctors. One of the stipulations is that all divers must have a chest X-ray which must be renewed at intervals depending on the diver's age.

The medical risks associated with diving are much higher than with most outdoor activities. Existing ear and sinus problems can be greatly worsened by the effect of water pressure. Asthmatics are not necessarily barred from diving but should be assessed individually. No school diving club can operate without a recognized qualified diving instructor and all equipment, including compressors, must be maintained to a very high standard.

Full details of equipment and diving safety may be obtained from the British Sub-Aqua Club.

Caving

Dry caves may require only the simplest of equipment: old boots, overalls, helmet and lamp. However, longer, wetter caves may require wetsuits, and a safety kit containing first aid equipment, survival bag, candles, waterproof matches, spare torches and an emergency ration pack should always be carried in a waterproof box. Simple accidents can produce major problems in caves, and safety ropes should always be used for ladder work and abseiling. Free diving sumps should have a hand line and an adult at each end. The leader should know the strength of his party and be aware of the problems of exhaustion in wet, cold conditions.

Sailing and windsurfing

The problems of our often intemperate climate apply particularly to these sports, in which careful attention to maintenance of body heat is important. Buoyancy aids or life jackets should always be worn and the difference of scale between lake and sea sailing should always be remembered. A party should obtain local information on wind and tide before sailing or surfing at sea.

Skiing

Many accidents are caused by poorly fitted equipment, and the leader of the party should make sure that boots, bindings and skis are suitable and correctly adjusted. Pre-ski training is essential, but since few pupils will carry out the gymnastic exercises for this adequately, it is better to use artificial ski slopes when possible to prepare their limbs for the snow.

Clothing is important and should allow for changes in conditions. Snow glasses or goggles are essential and three or four thin layers of vest, thin shirt, sweater and ski jacket allow for variations in temperature. A hat is of practical value. The leader of a skiing party should be aware of the problems of sunburn and make sure that all members of the party use sunburn creams adequately.

Addresses

British Mountaineering Council, Crawford House, Precinct Centre, Booth Street East, Manchester M13 9RZ
Telephone: 061-273 5835

British Canoe Union, Flexel House, 45/47 High Street, Addlestone, Surrey

British Sub-Aqua Club, 70 Brompton Road, London SW3 1HA
Telephone: 01-584 7163/4

National Caving Association, c/o Whernside Cave and Fell Centre, Dent, Sedbergh, Cumbria
Telephone: 05875 213

British Schools Exploring Society, C/o Royal Geographical Society,
1 Kensington Gore, London SW7 2AR
Telephone: 01-584 0710

Young Explorers' Trust C/o Royal Geographical Society,
1 Kensington Gore, London SW7 2AR
Telephone: 01-589 9724

Further reading

Pugh, L. G. C. E. (1966). Accidental hypothermia in walkers,
climbers and campers. *Br. Med. J.*, 1, 123
Steele, P. (1976). *Medical Care for Mountain Climbers*. (London:
William Heinemann Medical Books)
Wilkinson, J. A. (ed.) (1975). *Medicine for Mountaineering*. (Seat-
tle: The Mountaineers)

Accident prevention

The following aspects of safety at school are dealt with in more
details in the DES booklets [1-5].

Fire precautions

The design of buildings plays an important part in fire prevention,
and inspections should be made periodically by the chief fire officer.
Fire drills to practise evacuation of buildings should be carried out
regularly and fire extinguishers should be maintained and
recharged according to the manufacturers' instructions.

Precautions in the use of electricity

All electrical apparatus must be properly wired to a mains plug.
Particular care is required over electrical musical instruments, as
fatalities have been caused by the failure of the earth or trans-
former. Electric guitars and sound reproduction apparatus should
be forbidden until inspected and approved by a qualified electri-
cian.

Road safety

Road safety is an important part of nursery and primary school teaching. Bicycle training and testing are organized by the Royal Society for Prevention of Accidents. All cyclists should know the Highway Code, and bicycles should be maintained in good order, reinforced by inspection if necessary. Motor vehicle instruction should be given only by qualified instructors, and pupils under instruction must have their parents' written consent.

Science laboratories

The DES booklet *Safety in Science Laboratories*[2] is essential reading. It is worth mentioning the commonest laboratory accident which depends on immediate first aid to prevent permanent damage: the splashing of hot acid or alkali in the eyes. All science teachers should be familiar with the need for instant flooding with copious cold water in these cases.

School premises

Many accidents are caused by the use of plate glass in swing doors and partitions. Wherever possible reinforced glass should be used. In cloakrooms and bathrooms roller towels should be avoided as they have caused occasional fatal accidents by strangulation in younger children.

Physical education

Sports injuries were dealt with in Chapter 7. Other aspects are covered in *Safety in Physical Education*[4] which reproduces the rules of the Amateur Athletic Association on safety. Failure to follow these rules continues to result in fatal accidents particularly in throwing events.

References

1. Department of Education and Science (1972). *Safety in Outdoor Pursuits*. DES Safety Series No. 1. (London: HMSO)
2. Department of Education and Science (1976). *Safety in Science Laboratories*. 2nd Edn. DES Safety Series No. 2. (London: HMSO)
3. Department of Education and Science (1973). *Safety in Practical Departments*. DES Safety Series No. 3. (London: HMSO)
4. Department of Education and Science (1975). *Safety in Physical Education*. 2nd Edn. DES Safety Series No. 4. (London: HMSO)
5. Department of Education and Science (1979). *Safety at School: General Advice*. 2nd Edn. DES Safety Series No. 6. (London: HMSO)

CHAPTER 9

COMMUNICABLE DISEASES

Respiratory infections

The common cold

The common cold is an acute respiratory illness in which the brunt of the infection falls on the mucous membrane of the upper respiratory tract, leading to rhinorrhoea, nasal obstruction, sneezing and a dry cough. The duration is usually about a week. The majority of common colds are caused by rhinoviruses, of which there are over 100 distinct serotypes. Other viruses concerned to a lesser extent in the causation of colds are coronaviruses and enteroviruses.

Diagnosis

Diagnosis is largely on clinical grounds as the virus is isolated with difficulty from nasal washings.

Infection and transmission

Experimentally the common cold has been found surprisingly difficult to transmit from one person to another[1]. Infection appears to be mainly by hand-to-hand contact.

Incubation period

1–4 days.

Period of communicability

Colds are most commonly communicated in the active stage, but may be transmitted up to 8 days from onset.

Immunity

Immunity is type-specific and prolonged, but there is no cross-immunity between strains of rhinovirus.

Prevention

There is no known method of preventing common colds, despite unsubstantiated claims of the efficacy of vitamin C in large doses.

Treatment

Treatment is purely symptomatic. There is no place for the use of antibiotics.

Return to school

Children with heavy nasal discharge or complications should be kept at home or in the sanatorium until clear. Swimming, especially if the individual has a history of otitis media, should be restricted. Young children should not undertake heavy physical exertion until full recovery.

Streptococcal pharyngitis and tonsillitis

Sore throats may be caused by a variety of viruses or by the beta haemolytic streptococcus. Diphtheria (p. 159) is now a rarity. Human streptococcal throat infection is nearly always caused by strains of Lancefield Group A. Although other groups may be isolated from throat swabs they are seldom pathogenic. The symptoms of streptococcal pharyngitis or tonsillitis are severe sore throat with pain on swallowing, and usually a constitutional illness with high fever. The cervical lymph nodes are often enlarged. Uncommonly, an erythrogenic strain of the organism produces a scarlatiniform rash and strawberry tongue, on the basis of which scarlet fever, a notifiable disease, is diagnosed. Occasionally a peritonsillar abscess (quinsy) develops.

Some epidemic strains of streptococci cause acute

glomerulonephritis and rheumatic fever, but these have become rare.

Diagnosis

The diagnosis is made on the clinical appearance of redness of the throat in the case of pharyngitis, and enlargement of the tonsils with a purulent, cheesy exudate oozing from the tonsillar crypts in the case of tonsillitis, supported by isolation of a group A streptococcus from the throat swab. Typing of the streptococcus will show whether the strain is one associated with rash, rheumatic fever or nephritis.

Infection and transmission

Transmission is by droplet infection and may be from symptomless carriers. Nasal and salivary carriers are more infectious than faucial carriers. Streptococcal infection has occasionally been transmitted by unpasteurized milk.

Incubation period

The incubation period is short, usually 2–3 days, but may be from 1 to 6 days.

Period of communicability

Adequate antibiotic treatment will render patients virtually non-infectious within 24 hours. A carrier-state may persist, however, and this is sometimes extremely troublesome in boarding schools.

Prevention

Streptococcal infections may be prevented by long-term oral penicillin or erythromycin (250 mg b.d.) in those in whom they would constitute a special risk. In practice this means those who have had an attack of rheumatic fever.

The risk of milk-borne streptococcal infection is eliminated by pasteurization.

Methods of control

The patient with a suspected streptococcal infection should be kept away from school and isolated in a single room for the first 24 hours of antibiotic treatment.

An extensive outbreak in a school can cause considerable ill health and disruption, and may continue for longer than an influenza outbreak. It may then be advisable, with the co-operation of the Public Health Laboratory Service (see Appendix A, pp. 182–6) to undertake mass swabbing. Salivary and nasal swabs are the most relevant in the detection of contacts, who should then be treated with penicillin or erythromycin to eliminate the infection. In nasal carriers, insufflation of sulphonamide powder has been used successfully.

Treatment

The streptococcus invariably responds dramatically to penicillin, and no other antibiotic is indicated except erythromycin for those who are allergic to penicillin. As the majority of sore throats are self-limiting virus infections, the doctor has to exercise judgement in deciding whether to use antibiotics in an individual case. It is always wise to take a throat swab and act on the result, but a decision must be made on clinical grounds while the swab is being cultured. It is generally agreed that all cases of streptococcal throat infection should be treated with antibiotics because of their rapid response and risk of complications; but there is less unanimity about what to do in individual cases of sore throat. Most would agree that if there is constitutional upset, an acutely red pharynx, tonsillitis, lymphadenopathy, otitis media or a scarlatiniform rash, treatment should begin at once. Oral penicillin V (250 mg q.d.s. before meals) is usually sufficient, but intramuscular penicillin can be used in the acutely ill, and an injection of Triplopen can be valuable when patient compliance is in doubt. If the throat swab is negative oral penicillin can be discontinued, but if it is positive it is important to continue for 10 days, as relapse is common. On no account should ampicillin or amoxycillin be given, because of the likelihood of provoking an unpleasant rash if the infection should prove to be infectious mononucleosis (p. 154).

Return to school

The patient can return to school on clinical recovery.

Adenovirus infections

There are 33 serotypes of adenovirus, causing several different clinical syndromes:

(a) *Pharyngitis,* an acute febrile illness with enlargement of the regional lymph nodes. The throat is red and oedematous and there may be follicular exudate. The nose is often involved and develops a thick mucopurulent discharge. In spite of the fever, constitutional symptoms are not very severe and convalescence is rapid.

(b) *Pharyngoconjunctival fever,* usually caused by Type 3 or Type 7. Epidemics occur in schools from time to time. It is characterized by fever, sore throat, swelling of the cervical lymph nodes, and coryza-like symptoms, followed by conjunctivitis with purulent discharge and photophobia. The conjunctivitis may be unilateral and may occur in the absence of other symptoms. Pharyngoconjunctival fever is commoner in summer than winter.

(c) *Acute respiratory disease.* The throat is again involved but the glandular enlargement is not so marked and the lower respiratory tract is invaded, sometimes with the development of pneumonia. (see p. 134).

(d) *Epidemic kerato-conjunctivitis.* This is a more general and chronic condition affecting the eyes alone and occurs in small epidemics. Transmission may be by dust with consequent conjunctival damage or by contamination with ophthalmic instruments or droppers. It is generally due to Type 8 adenovirus.

The transmission of adenovirus infections is by droplet infection, and the diagnosis can be made by isolation of the virus from throat swabs and eye swabs. The incubation period is about a week, and immunity is type-specific and probably long-lasting. Isolation is not necessary and no specific treatment is effective.

Croup

Croup is the result of airway obstruction due to respiratory infection in young children. It may lead to a brassy cough and inspiratory stridor. It is most commonly due to laryngo-tracheo-bronchitis, often caused by parainfluenza or respiratory syncytial virus (RSV) infection. Rarer but more dangerous, acute epiglottitis occurs in a slightly older age group, from 2 to 6 years, and is invariably due to *H. influenzae* type B.

Laryngo-tracheo-bronchitis is best treated with bed rest and steam. If acute epiglottitis is suspected – as suggested by the sudden onset and toxicity in the child – examination of the pharynx is contraindicated as it may cause obstruction. Urgent hospital admission is advisable.

Otitis media

Probably only about a quarter of cases of otitis media are bacterial in origin. In children under the age of 4 years *H. influenzae* is the commonest bacterium involved. Over that age pneumococci are commonest. The complications of acute otitis media include chronic discharging otitis media, deafness, and more rarely mastoiditis and meningitis, so the use of antibiotics in all cases has some justification. Ampicillin is effective against *H. influenzae,* penicillin and erythromycin against pneumococci, and cotrimoxazole is usually effective against both organisms.

Bronchitis and bronchiolitis

Bronchitis may be defined as an infection of the lower respiratory tract with adventitious sounds but no clinical or radiological signs of consolidation. It is usually of viral aetiology. The symptoms are cough and fever. In children with recurrent attacks, the diagnosis of asthma should be considered (see Chapter 5, p. 77).

Bronchiolitis is an epidemic disease of infants, frequently due to RSV.

Pneumonia

Pneumonia is an acute infection of the lungs with radiological signs of consolidation. Classical lobar pneumonia is uncommon and can cause diagnostic difficulties due to the high fever and prostration which may occur before the development of clinical signs in the lungs. *Strep. pneumoniae* is the commonest cause, and penicillin is therefore the drug of choice.

Bronchopneumonia, with its more diffuse and patchy consolidation, may be caused by bacterial or viral infection with approximately equal frequency. It may occur as a secondary infection after influenza. The bacteria most commonly involved are *Strep. pneumoniae, Mycoplasma pneumoniae* and staphylococci. Viruses include RSV, parainfluenza, adenovirus and influenza.

Mycoplasma pneumoniae

Infection with *Mycoplasma pneumoniae* has an insidious onset, with fever and malaise preceding cough, which may not at first be accompanied by adventitious sounds in the lungs. Radiological changes are often more widespread than the clinical signs suggest, and usually consist of soft miliary mottling. Bullous myringitis may accompany the infection.

The organism may be grown from throat swabs or sputum. The diagnosis can also be made serologically from paired sera. Immunity is probably long-lasting. Tetracycline and erythromycin are effective in *M. pneumoniae* infections but have to be given for several days after the temperature has returned to normal.

Staphylococcal pneumonia

Staphylococci are an uncommon cause of pneumonia, but may be implicated as secondary invaders in influenza. The infection may then be fulminating, requiring intravenous treatment with hydrocortisone and antibiotics such as cloxacillin which are effective against penicillinase-producing staphylococci. Cloxacillin should be given until sensitivity results are received from the laboratory.

Respiratory syncytial virus (RSV)

RSV causes acute bronchiolitis and pneumonia in infants and young children. The infection also occurs in older children and adults, who may have mild infections of the common cold type, but the more severe illness with constitutional upset and lower respiratory tract involvement can also occur in these groups. Small epidemics occur in winter.

Parainfluenza infections

These infections are more severe than rhinovirus illnesses, but are not generally as severe as influenzal infections. The symptoms range from common colds and laryngitis to severe laryngo-tracheo-bronchitis (see p. 133) and pneumonia. In most cases fever does not exceed 38°C and lasts only 2–3 days; nasal discharge, cough and hoarseness are prominent. In more severe cases the signs of obstructive laryngitis or lower respiratory tract infection predominate.

Diagnosis is by isolation of the virus from throat or nose swabs or by demonstration of a rise in titre in paired sera.

Q fever

Q fever is caused by *Coxiella burneti,* and is carried by many insects, ticks and animals. The main reservoir in the UK is probably cattle and sheep, and occasional outbreaks are reported due to airborne spread or unpasteurized milk[2]. The commonest clinical presentation is pyrexia of unknown origin, which may be accompanied by a bewildering array of syndromes including atypical pneumonia and endocarditis. Treatment is with tetracycline.

Ornithosis and psittacosis

Ornithosis is an infection caused by Chlamydia B organisms, transmitted by birds. Psittacosis is the term used for disease transmitted by the parrot and budgerigar families. Clinically there is atypical pneumonia or milder respiratory infection. Treatment is with tetracycline.

Legionnaire's disease

Legionnaire's disease is a bacterial pneumonia which particularly affects elderly men with impaired respiratory function, and tends to occur in airborne outbreaks. It has not as yet been reported in schools.

Influenza

Influenza is a respiratory infection caused by influenza A or B virus (influenza C is rarely isolated from ill patients, and probably causes inapparent infections). Influenza A also affects many animals and birds, while influenza B appears to infect man only. Both can cause very large outbreaks in schools, and are unique in their capacity for antigenic variation. The surface antigens which undergo continual minor changes (antigen drift) and occasional major alterations (antigenic shift) are haemagglutinin and neuraminidase. The subtypes of influenza A are classified according to these surface anti-gens. H_1N_1, for example is the name given to the strain which first appeared in 1947 and reappeared in 1978. The massive epidemics of 1957 occurred after a change in both haemagglutinin and neuraminidase, and this virus was named H_2N_2. The next shift in 1968 involved haemagglutinin only, so the strain was called H_3N_2.

Symptoms

Influenza A and B are clinically indistinguishable. There is an acute febrile illness, generally with sudden onset and considerable con-stitutional symptoms and prostration. The conjunctivae and fauces show an early non-oedematous flushing and the respiratory tract, especially the trachea, is soon involved. The nose may also be inflamed and excoriated and sore throat may be complained of, although inflammation is slight. At the height of the illness, which is sometimes biphasic, prostration and constitutional distress may occur. In the average case fever, which may rise to 40°C, lasts for $2\frac{1}{2}$ days.

Mild cases of infection occur, and serological studies have shown that in any outbreak there is a considerable number of symptomless cases.

Complications

Pneumonia is an important complication. The dangerous fulminat-ing type which causes occasional deaths in schoolchildren may be due to overwhelming infection with the influenza virus itself or to staphylococcal secondary infection (see p. 135). Secondary bron-chopneumonia due to *Strep. pneumoniae* occurs more commonly. *H. influenzae* and haemolytic streptococci are other secondary invaders.

Reye's syndrome is a rare complication of influenza and some other virus infections. It consists of encephalopathy and fatty degeneration of the liver, and has a high mortality rate.

Diagnosis

The virus can be isolated from throat swabs or by special techniques using nasal aspirate which can provide evidence of the infecting virus in 3 hours. Retrospective diagnosis can be made by serological tests on acute and convalescent sera.

Table 4 Principal respiratory pathogens and syndromes

Agent	Illness	Notes
Rhinoviruses	Common colds, tracheitis and bronchitis	Over 100 serotypes
Parainfluenza viruses	Common colds and LRT infection, including pneumonia; in young children, laryngitis and croup (Types I and II).	Types I to IV
Influenza viruses types A and B	Epidemic influenza, LRT infections, including pneumonia. Some mild illnesses.	Major changes in antigens with Type A. Type B is more stable.
Respiratory syncytial virus (RSV)	Bronchitis, bronchiolitis and pneumonia. URT infection in older individuals.	A single unchanging type.
Coronaviruses	Common colds	
Adenoviruses	Predominantly cause pharyngitis, but also LRT infections, including pneumonia. Pharyngo-conjunctivitis.	33 serotypes. Endemic Types 1, 2, 3, 5, 6, 7. Epidemic Types 3, 4, 7, 14.
Coxsackie A viruses	Pharyngitis, herpangina; hand, foot and mouth disease.	24 serotypes. Also cause meningitis.
Coxsackie B viruses	Pharyngitis, Bornholm disease.	Six serotypes. Also cause meningitis and myocarditis.
Echoviruses	Pharyngitis, sometimes with rash (Types 9 and 10.) Common colds (Types 11, 20 and 28)	34 serotypes. Also cause meningitis.

Organism	Disease	Notes
Herpes simplex virus	Recurrent 'cold sores'. Primary infection usually produces stomatitis (Type I). Herpes genitalis (Type II).	Two serotypes. Rarely nervous system infection, keratitis or Kaposi's varicelliform eruption (Type I): severe neonatal generalized infection (Type II).
Epstein–Barr virus (EBV)	Infectious mononucleosis	Associated with Burkitt's lymphoma
Strep. pyogenes (Haemolytic streptococcus group A)	Pharyngitis, tonsillitis	Numerous serotypes. Nephritis (especially Type 12), rheumatic fever and chorea are rare sequelae
Strep. pneumoniae	Lobar pneumonia	80 serotypes. Also meningitis, pericarditis and other suppurative foci
Haemophilus influenzae	Croup, epiglottitis in infants, pneumonia, sinusitis	Also meningitis
Mycoplasma pneumoniae	LRT, especially pneumonia, milder URT infections	Bullous myringitis
Staphylococcus pyogenes	Pneumonia by secondary infection, sinusitis	Also other purulent lesions
Coxiella burneti	Pneumonia, febrile illness (Q fever)	Sometimes chronic. Reservoir of infection in farm animals
Chlamydia B	LRT infection and pneumonia. Also mild infections (Ornithosis and psittacosis)	Reservoir of infection in birds
Klebsiella pneumoniae	Pneumonia	Pulmonary abscess formation

URT: upper respiratory tract; LRT: lower respiratory tract.

Incubation period

2–3 days.

Period of communicability

Influenza is very readily transmitted to those who are susceptible to the epidemic strain. Communicability is probably greatest in the prodromal phase and lasts not more than 3 days from onset.

Immunity

Immunity is type-specific but is bedevilled by antigenic changes in the virus. Infection with one subtype of influenza A (e.g. H_3N_2) or with influenza B provides lasting immunity against the infecting strain and minor degrees of antigenic drift, but when the surface antigens have become sufficiently different from the parent strain, the patient may be susceptible to the new virus. Reinfection with the H_1N_1 strain appears to occur more readily in schoolchildren than with other strains.

Prevalence

Influenza usually occurs in epidemics in which a high proportion of the susceptible community is infected within 2 or 3 weeks of the first case. Influenza A epidemics occur more often than influenza B epidemics. The latter are mostly confined to schools and other institutions, tending to occur in 3–5 year cycles. Outbreaks usually occur between the months of December and April.

Prevention

The place of influenza vaccination in schools is controversial, and is dealt with in Chapter 3 (p. 43).

Amantadine is effective in the prevention of influenza A, but not influenza B, and has sometimes been used with advantage in school populations[3].

Treatment

There is no specific treatment, but secondary bacterial infections need to be treated with the appropriate antibiotic.

Return to school

In a boarding school epidemic with pressure on sanatorium accommodation, it is often necessary for pupils to return to school after the fever has settled. This causes no harm, so long as it is recognized that there may be some debility in the convalescent period. Sport should not be resumed for at least a week after recovery (see also p. 102).

The principal agents responsible for respiratory infections are listed in Table 4 together with their clinical effects and other characteristics.

The exanthemata

Measles

Measles is an infectious disease caused by a paramyxovirus and characterized by fever, respiratory symptoms, conjunctivitis and a dusky red blotchy macular rash. It is a notifiable disease which could become a rarity if vaccination policy were pursued as enthusiastically as in the USA.

Symptoms

A particularly troublesome dry cough develops associated with coryza and considerable fever. The conjunctivae are infected, as is the buccal mucosa, where Koplik's spots appear early and are pathognomonic. They consist of tiny white spots (likened to salt grains) on a red base. After about 4 days the rash appears, at first on the head and neck. During the following 48 hours it spreads to involve the trunk and limbs. The eruption is at first sparse but as further spots appear it becomes blotchy and confluent. During the eruptive stage the child remains miserable, nothing alleviating the cough satisfactorily. A day later dramatic improvement occurs. The rash begins to fade, the fever subsides and the cough is no longer distressing. Complications are not common in an otherwise healthy child but should be suspected when improvement does not occur in this way. They include otitis media, bronchopneumonia, purulent conjunctivitis and, very rarely, encephalitis. Children who have been immunized not uncommonly develop the disease though the symptoms may be relatively mild.

Diagnosis

The diagnosis may be overlooked in the catarrhal stage unless the buccal mucosa is carefully examined. Where a rash is present confusion may arise with a variety of common diseases, notably rubella and scarlet fever. Echoviruses and Coxsackie viruses may also cause maculopapular rashes. In roseola infantum the sick infant's condition improves dramatically with the appearance of the rash, a feature quite unlike measles. Erythema infectiosum (fifth disease) is a mild non-febrile erythematous eruption occurring in epidemics in children and causing a characteristic 'slapped cheek' appearance. Drug rashes may cause difficulties particularly those due to ampicillin and co-trimoxazole.

Laboratory diagnosis can be made by isolation of the appropriate virus from a swab taken from the nasopharynx early in the infection. Serological tests are also available. These procedures are indicated only where clinical doubt remains and where an exact diagnosis is particularly important.

Infection and transmission

This is by direct contact with a patient.

Incubation period

The incubation period is 10–15 days, usually 10 days from exposure to the onset of illness, and 14 days to the development of the rash.

Period of communicability

This is from the day before the development of symptoms until the disappearance of the rash.

Immunity

One attack normally confers immunity.

Prevention

Measles vaccine prevents the disease in approximately 95% of those vaccinated. When the disease does occur in a vaccinated child it is usually mild (see Chapter 3, p. 41).

During an outbreak, measles vaccine given to susceptible contacts is effective early in the incubation period. Human pooled immunoglobulin can be used up to a late stage in patients at special risk.

Treatment

There is no specific treatment for measles. Antibiotics are indicated only to treat secondary infection but may be used prophylactically in those children who are unduly susceptible to any of the common complications.

Return to school

Pupils may return to school on clinical recovery, provided this is not earlier than 7 days after the onset of the rash.

Rubella (German measles)

Rubella is an infectious disease caused by a virus. It is normally a very mild illness in which a generalized pink macular rash is associated with enlarged tender suboccipital glands. The importance of rubella lies in the risk of the congenital rubella syndrome.

Symptoms

Malaise with low fever and minimal respiratory symptoms develop simultaneously with the rash. This spreads rapidly from the head and neck downwards. Joint pains and swelling may occur, especially in adult women. The rash fades and recovery takes place in 4 or 5 days. Occasionally infection may occur without a rash. Complications are rare with the exception of congenital rubella. This affects some infants born to mothers who have contracted clinical or subclinical rubella during the first 4 months of pregnancy. 10–15% of these infants may have cataracts, cardiac abnormalities, deafness, mental deficiency or microcephaly. The infant may be born with the expanded rubella syndrome which is due to active infection with the rubella virus. The danger of cross-infection may persist for a year. Features of this infection include failure to gain weight, jaundice, anaemia and a rash. There may be enlargement of the liver and spleen, generalized lymphadenopathy, thrombocytopenic purpura and myocarditis. Termination of pregnancy should be considered where infection of the mother (proved serologically) has occurred.

Diagnosis

Clinical diagnosis is far from reliable, as the rash may easily be confused with many others.

Diagnosis can be confirmed by virus isolation and serology. It is of greatest importance in women in early pregnancy, when rubella-specific IgM is the most helpful indication of recent infection.

Infection and transmission

This is by droplet infection.

Incubation period

14–21 days, usually 18.

Period of communicability

This is a few days before the onset of the symptoms and for 4 days after the appearance of the rash.

Immunity

One attack usually confers lifelong immunity. The common history of apparent multiple attacks simply emphasizes the difficulty of accurate clinical diagnosis.

Prevention

Rubella can be prevented by a live vaccine, which is offered to girls between the ages of 10 and 13. This is fully dealt with in Chapter 3 (p. 41).

Parents and staff should be informed when cases occur in a school, and the opportunity taken of reminding them of the congenital rubella syndrome and how it can be prevented.

Treatment

There is no specific treatment.

Return to school

Pupils can return as soon as they are well. It can be argued that isolation is against the interests of uninfected children, but if the school insists on exclusion it should be until 4 days after the appearance of the rash.

Chickenpox (Varicella)

Chickenpox is an acute infectious disease with fever, constitutional symptoms and a vesicular rash due to the varicella-zoster virus.

Symptoms

The rash is distributed centripetally and the flexures are involved. Sparse rashes are common. The symptoms tend to be more severe in older patients. Maculopapules last a few hours before becoming vesicles, then pustules last 3 or 4 days and finally form scabs. Successive crops may be present at the same time, producing a pleomorphic rash. Vesico-ulcerative lesions of the mouth appear early and are sparse. Varicella pneumonia, encephalitis and haemorrhagic chickenpox are rare but serious complications.

Diagnosis

The diagnosis seldom presents difficulty, as the vesicles are quite characteristic.

Infection and transmission

The spread is mainly by droplet infection, but the early skin lesions are also infectious. Contact with herpes zoster may cause chickenpox in susceptible children, but the infectivity is not great.

Incubation period

Between 11 and 20 days, most commonly about 16 days.

Period of communicability

Chickenpox is probably infectious from several days before the rash until the last spot has crusted.

Immunity

One attack confers permanent immunity. An attack of chickenpox does not confer immunity against herpes zoster, which occurs with the reactivation of the varicella-zoster virus in a dorsal sensory ganglion.

Prevention

Work is proceeding on a vaccine which may in the future prevent chickenpox and herpes zoster.

Treatment

Local application of calamine reduces the irritation of the chicken-pox spots. Oral antihistamines may also be helpful.

Return to school

Patients may return to school 6 days after the appearance of the rash, unless heavily scabbed.

Herpes zoster (shingles)

Herpes zoster is usually due to reactivation of the varicella-zoster virus lying dormant in a dorsal root ganglion since an attack of chickenpox years previously. More rarely it develops as a result of direct exposure to chickenpox. It is characterized by a unilateral vesicular eruption confined to the distribution of the corresponding sensory nerve.

Symptoms

Adults are affected more frequently than children. The eruption is preceded by pain in the same area for several days. Patches of erythema develop in which crops of vesicles soon appear. The vesicles dry up and form scabs in a week or 10 days. Considerable scarring may be left when the scabs have separated. The intercostal nerves are most frequently involved, but the eruption may occur anywhere on the body. The ophthalmic nerve may be affected and be followed by keratitis and iridocyclitis. Pain may persist for months after the eruption has disappeared, particularly in the elderly (postherpetic neuralgia). Rarely motor nuclei close to the affected sensory ganglion are also involved, causing local paralysis. Herpes of the external auditory meatus and palate associated with facial paralysis constitutes the Ramsay–Hunt syndrome.

Incubation period

The incubation period when there is direct infection is 3–7 days.

Period of communicability

Herpes zoster is not very infectious, but child contacts may develop chickenpox, and there is some evidence for case-to-case spread. The period of communicability is likely to be similar to chickenpox: until 6 days after the appearance of the rash.

Immunity

One attack confers permanent immunity with rare exceptions.

Treatment

Specific treatment with idoxuridine paint reduces the duration of the symptoms and the incidence of postherpetic neuralgia. Pain should be treated with analgesics.

Return to school

The disease is often mild in children, and they need not necessarily be excluded from school in view of the low infectivity of herpes zoster. In more severe cases, they can return to school on clinical recovery.

Herpes simplex

There are two serotypes of this common virus infection which causes a vesicular eruption on the skin or mucous membrane preceded by an itching or burning sensation. Type I causes mucocutaneous lesions and occasionally encephalitis. Type II causes herpes genitalis (see p. 171) and neonatal herpes infections from contact with the mother's genital tract during birth.

The commonest presentation of primary infection with Type I in childhood is ulcerative stomatitis. It can also present as keratitis of the eyes and dendritic ulceration, or as 'scrumpox'. This is more prolonged and severe than bacterial impetigo, often with marked cervical lymphadenopathy and fever, and can be transmitted by the close contact of the Rugby scrum. With fewer people developing primary infections in childhood, it is possible that this type of 'scrumpox' is becoming commoner.

Recurrent herpes simplex infection is the cause of 'cold sores' or herpes labialis. The virus lies dormant following a primary infection and when reactivated produces vesicular lesions around the lips. Herpetic eruptions are often associated with the common cold, and with influenza and pneumonia; they occur after trauma, exposure to sunlight or cold and during menstruation or in emotional upsets. In eczematous subjects, infection may cause eczema herpeticum (Kaposi's varicelliform eruption).

Diagnosis

Diagnosis is on clinical grounds. It can be confirmed by electron microscopy of vesicle fluid and by culture of the virus. A serological response can also be demonstrated.

Incubation period

4–5 days.

Period of communicability

7–10 days.

Prevention

Anybody with a 'scrumpox' rash should not play Rugby football.

Treatment

Antiviral agents such as idoxuridine and acyclovir are effective against herpes simplex and can be used if the symptoms are severe. They are expensive, however, and simple antiseptics such as Eusol or povidine–iodine are usually all that is necessary for cold sores.

Smallpox (Variola)

Smallpox was a dangerous illness once included in the differential diagnosis of chickenpox. The world has been free of the disease since 1979.

Virus infections

Mumps

Mumps is an acute infectious disease spread by droplet infection and caused by a virus. It is characterized by painful swelling of the salivary glands.

Symptoms

Fever and headache develop in association with swelling of one or more of the salivary glands, the parotids being the most commonly affected. The symptoms gradually subside in about a week. Orchitis is a rare complication before puberty but occurs in a proportion of males after puberty. It may be followed by a degree of testicular atrophy but infertility is rare. Lymphocytic meningitis and meningoencephalitis may also occur as may permanent deafness, pancreatitis and oophoritis. Rarely, a complication may occur without involvement of the salivary glands.

Diagnosis

Lymphadenitis from tonsillitis or infectious mononucleosis must be differentiated from the salivary gland swelling of mumps. Recurrent parotitis is frequently mistaken for mumps in the first attack. Torsion of the testis must be excluded before diagnosing orchitis. Serological diagnosis is possible but seldom necessary, and the serum amylase is raised in 90% of cases with clinical parotitis.

Incubation period

Outside limits of 12–26 days are usually quoted, but the incubation period is commonly from 16 to 18 days.

Period of communicability

Mumps, which has low infectivity, is communicable from a few days before the onset of symptoms until about 4 days after the onset of salivary gland swelling.

Immunity

One attack confers lifelong immunity. Infection often causes inapparent or subclinical illness, and serological studies show that at least 90% of the population are immune by the age of 14.

Prevention

Spread of the disease may be prevented by isolation of cases during the acute illness. An effective live vaccine is available. In the UK it is not recommended as a routine measure, but might well be offered to boys who are found to be seronegative at the onset of puberty, in view of the possible complication of orchitis.

Treatment

There is no specific treatment for mumps. The acute pain of orchitis may be helped by the use of a suspensory bandage. Prednisolone in a dose of 10 mg 4 times a day has been found useful.

Return to school

Pupils may return to school on recovery.

Hepatitis A

Hepatitis A is an acute inflammatory disease of the liver caused by a picornavirus. It is transmitted by the faecal–oral route, and is predominantly a disease of young people, often associated with travel abroad or consumption of raw shellfish. Epidemics sometimes occur in closed communities. A few days prior to the appearance of clinical signs, the patient may have a mild febrile illness with anorexia and malaise. This is usually followed by nausea, vomiting, fever and pain in the upper right quadrant of the abdomen. Simultaneously, or a few days later, jaundice with bile in the urine will appear followed by pruritis and bradycardia. In an epidemic many mild cases fail to develop jaundice. The liver is usually enlarged and tender. In the majority of cases the disease is mild and resolves spontaneously in 3–6 weeks.

Diagnosis

Hepatitis A can be diagnosed serologically from a single blood specimen. Blood should be sent to the laboratory for liver function tests and these should be repeated to follow progress (see p. 25 for special precautions in taking blood). The differential diagnosis of jaundice is large, and includes infectious mononucleosis, cytomegalovirus infections, toxoplasmosis and Weil's disease.

Incubation period

The incubation period varies between 15 and 40 days.

Period of communicability

This is from before the onset of clinical signs for at least 3–4 weeks. In isolated cases a carrier state may persist for years.

Immunity

Relapses occasionally occur within 2 months of the original illness. Second attacks later than this are rare.

Prevention

Patients should be isolated at home or in the school sanatorium. Infective hepatitis is a notifiable disease. Human gamma globulin will provide short-term protection for travellers likely to be at high risk (see Chapter 3, p. 47).

Treatment

There is no specific treatment.

Return to school

Pupils may return to school when clinically recovered. However, liver function tests may not return to normal for several months and convalescence may be prolonged, with some restriction necessary on sporting activities.

Hepatitis B

Hepatitis B is caused by a more complex virus, and the disease and its aftermath are generally more serious than hepatitis A. It affects all ages, has a long incubation period, 40–180 days, and is transmitted by infected blood or blood products from a sufferer or carrier, or by sexual contact, as the virus is present in many body secretions. It is a particular risk in self-injecting drug abusers, and can be transmitted in tattooing and acupuncture. Particular care is necessary in taking and handling blood specimens where there is a possibility of hepatitis B (see Chapter 2, p. 25). Hepatitis B vaccine is discussed in Chapter 3, p 44.

Non-A non-B hepatitis

Some cases of blood-transmitted hepatitis are found to be caused by neither hepatitis A nor hepatitis B virus. In our present state of knowledge they are called non-A non-B hepatitis.

Poliomyelitis

Poliomyelitis is an acute virus infection in which about half the patients have a minor prodromal illness. The major illness which may follow a few days later ranges from aseptic meningitis without paralysis to extensive flaccid paralysis. The causative organism is an enterovirus of which there are three distinct serotypes. As a result of immunization (see Chapter 3, p. 40), poliomyelitis is now a rare disease in the UK, where it is a notifiable disease, but is still prevalent in most tropical countries.

Enterovirus infections (Coxsackie and echo viruses)

In addition to the three polio viruses, the enteroviruses consist of Coxsackie A (24 serotypes), Coxsackie B (6 serotypes) and echo viruses (34 serotypes). They are spread by the faecal–oral route to infect the pharynx and alimentary tract. They may then cause a viraemia with further spread to other organs and especially the nervous system. They can all cause acute febrile illnesses with a variety of symptoms including meningism, myalgia, respiratory tract infection, glandular enlargement, mild diarrhoea or vomiting, and rashes. There are certain specific syndromes associated with different serotypes. These are:

(a) *Epidemic myalgia (Bornholm disease)* Coxsackie B viruses cause this febrile illness with severe stitch-like pains in thoracic, abdominal or limb muscles. Fever is present to 39°C, and a biphasic course is common. Complications include pleurisy, pericarditis and orchitis. Myocarditis may occur and infected infants may succumb to this. Differential diagnosis from intrathoracic or abdominal disease is, of course, crucial.

(b) *Lymphocytic meningitis* Most of the enteroviruses and mumps virus (see p. 149) can cause lymphocytic meningitis. The onset is usually sudden with headache, photophobia, vomiting and drowsiness. Neck stiffness is present. The main illness may follow a minor illness due to the same agent. In some cases a rash may occur. The CSF shows an increased cell count with a preponderance of lymphocytes but without visible organisms. (At the onset there may be a neutrophil excess.) The course of the illness is usually mild and short. Many transient mild cases occur, with little more than meningism. In epidemics other manifestations of infection with the same agent occur in the community.

(c)   *Hand, foot and mouth disease* Small, discrete vesicles about 0.5 mm in diameter with surrounding erythema occur on the hands and feet, both on the soles and palms and also on the sides of the fingers and toes. They also occur on the buccal mucous membrane and tongue, and cause soreness. The patient may be afebrile or have pharyngitis with fever. This illness is especially associated with Coxsackie virus A16 and is usually mild and short.

(d)   *Herpangina* This is also caused by Coxsackie A virus. It has an abrupt onset, with fever up to 40°C, sore throat and enlarged cervical glands. Small vesicles 1–2 mm in diameter on an erythematous base develop on the soft palate and fauces, and are followed by shallow ulcers. The lesions do not extend to the anterior part of the mouth. The illness lasts up to 4 days.

Diagnosis

Enterovirus infections can be diagnosed by isolation of the virus from the throat, faeces or CSF.

Incubation period

The incubation period for enterovirus infection is between 2 and 5 days.

Period of communicability

These illnesses are probably communicable during the acute phase, possibly longer when the virus continues to be excreted in the faeces.

Immunity

Immunity is type-specific and long lasting.

Prevention

Little can be done to prevent the spread of enterovirus infections, but cases of meningitis should be isolated during the acute illness, and care taken over personal hygiene and the disposal of excreta.

Treatment

There is no specific treatment.

Return to school

Pupils can return to school on recovery.

Infectious mononucleosis (glandular fever)

Infectious mononucleosis is caused by the Epstein–Barr virus (EBV). In young children infections are often mild and unrecognized, but those in the 15–25 year age group usually develop a more severe illness.

Symptoms

The onset is often gradual and ill-defined, with headache, malaise and fever. Soreness of the throat follows immediately, or within one or two days of onset, and is often severe. Within a few days, the patient may be very uncomfortable, with prostration, a fever as high as 40°C, grossly enlarged tonsils and a confluent white exudate covering the tonsillar area. There are frequently petechiae on the palate. The nasopharanx may be congested, with some oedema of the eyelids. Swallowing and respiration may be embarrassed. The cervical lymph nodes, especially in the posterior triangles, are enlarged and cause discomfort but are not very tender. Other lymph nodes, the liver and the spleen may also be enlarged. Illness and fever fluctuate for 7–10 days (exceptionally up to 3 weeks) and then all symptoms and signs gradually resolve. Convalescence may be slow, and the patient tires easily. Prolonged debility sometimes occurs, especially in girls, but less often than is popularly supposed. After the acute state, relapses do not occur, although second attacks after an interval of years are not unknown.

A variant includes fever and lymph node enlargement without throat abnormalities. Jaundice occurs in about 10% of cases. Biochemical tests of liver function indicate that this organ is affected in the majority of cases.

Complications

Complications are rare but include a rash which is usually faint and transient. However, a florid morbilliform rash may occur in up to 90% of cases treated with ampicillin and is directly due to the use of this drug. For this reason ampicillin and amoxycillin are contraindicated whenever there is a possibility of infectious mononucleosis.

Splenic rupture may rarely occur during the acute or convalescent stage. The spleen may be very friable and be damaged by examination. Urgent surgical treatment is, of course, indicated. Neurological complications also occur but are uncommon.

Diagnosis

An absolute mononucleosis with atypical lymphocytes develops. Heterophile antibodies to sheep's red blood cells develop in the majority of cases during the acute phase but are occasionally delayed until convalescence. The Paul–Bunnell test detects these antibodies, but a simpler variation, the monospot test, is now generally used. Antibodies to EB virus develop early in the infection and are already present when the illness appears, so they are of little value in routine diagnosis.

In its early stages the illness must be differentiated from streptococcal and other viral infections, but none of these cause the full clinical picture of infectious mononucleosis. Cytomegalovirus and *Toxoplasma gondii* infections, described below, can have close similarities but may be differentiated by a negative Paul–Bunnell test and confirmed by specific serological tests.

Incubation period

The incubation period is unknown, but is probably long, up to several weeks.

Period of communicability

It is believed that contact has to be close for the disease to be transmitted, and it is therefore popularly called 'the kissing disease', with no more than circumstantial evidence to prove it. The period of communicability is unknown, but is probably confined to the acute phase of the illness.

Immunity

Immunity is usually permanent after an attack but individuals may be immune by reason of silent or mild infection in earlier life. There have been several studies in the UK showing that the proportion of children of school age with EB virus antibody in their blood is about 35–40%; in university entrants it has been found to be 57%. This is in contrast to studies in children in developing countries, where EB virus infection has been found to occur in the first two years of life in 75–80% of children.

Treatment

There is no specific treatment, but symptomatic treatment is needed during the acute phase. Steroids may be necessary in cases with pharyngeal or respiratory obstruction. Ampicillin and amoxycillin are strongly contraindicated. Antibiotics are of no benefit in any case, but if treatment is to be given while awaiting laboratory differentiation between streptococcal tonsillitis and infectious mononucleosis, penicillin or erythromycin are the drugs of choice.

Return to school

Pupils should return to school after clinical recovery and a period of convalescence, which can in most cases be brief.

Cytomegalovirus infections

Infection with cytomegalovirus (CMV) is worldwide, and a large proportion of the adult population has antibodies. Although most infections are inapparent, the organism is important as it may cause severe damage or death to the fetus or neonate. In schoolchildren it causes a syndrome similar to infectious mononucleosis, with atypical lymphocytes and abnormal liver function tests. Lymphatic enlargement and throat infection are not as common as in the classical disease. The Paul–Bunnell and monospot tests are negative. Pneumonia and liver disease have been described in children and adults due to CMV infection. The diagnosis may be made from serological tests, particularly a raised IgM or an antibody rise in paired sera.

Toxoplasmosis

Although a protozoal, not a viral, disease, toxoplasmosis is best considered here because its commonest manifestation at school age is an infectious mononucleosis-like syndrome with a negative Paul–Bunnell test. The cervical lymph nodes are most often involved but the spleen is not usually palpable. Sore throat is not consistently present but the fever is generally slight and long lasting, so that the illness may pursue a protracted course for several months. More severe manifestations include choroidoretinitis, acute encephalitis and pneumonia. Like CMV infections, toxoplasmosis can cause profound damage to the fetus and neonate. Diagnosis is serological. The source of human infection is raw or undercooked meat or the faeces of domestic animals such as dogs or cats. Specific treatment is not necessary in uncomplicated glandular toxoplasmosis. In unusually severe or prolonged cases, spiramycin can be effective.

Bacterial infections

Streptococcal infections

Streptococci are among the most important bacteria causing illness in schoolchildren. They are dealt with in the sections on respiratory infections (p. 130) and skin infections (p. 172).

Staphylococcal infections

Numerous infections may be caused by staphylococci, the usual pathogenic staphylococcus being the coagulase positive *Staphylococcus aureus* of which there are many phage types. It is the one organism above all others which is liable to develop resistance to antibiotics. Most manifestations of staphylococcal infection are dealt with in the sections on respiratory infections (p. 135), intestinal infections (p. 163) and skin infections (p. 172). The one uncommon but important remaining staphylococcal infection is osteomyelitis.

Osteomyelitis occurs as a complication of septicaemia or local spread of sepsis, usually but not always due to staphylococci. The usual source is skin sepsis. The cardinal symptom is bone pain at the site of the infection, which is generally in the metaphysis of a long bone. The child is usually febrile with a leukocytosis and raised ESR, and tenderness can be elicited over the diseased bone. Early diagnosis is important, and is best made by blood culture as X-ray changes do not develop immediately. The prompt use of antibiotics such as flucloxacillin may make surgical drainage unnecessary, but an orthopaedic surgeon should be consulted at an early stage. If energetic treatment is not instituted, chronic infection may develop, with the ultimate need for operation to remove sequestrum. Septic arthritis may develop in an adjacent joint. There has been a slight resurgence in the incidence of osteomyelitis, and vigilance is necessary if the diagnosis is to be made promptly.

Acute bacterial meningitis

The commonest cause of acute bacterial meningitis is the meningococcus *(Neisseria meningitidis),* followed by the pneumococcus and *H. influenzae.* Numerous other organisms may be responsible for meningitis, such as streptococci and staphylococci, which are usually secondary to infections of the middle ear or paranasal sinuses. Other pyogenic forms due to *E. coli* and salmonellae are more common in infants, or may be secondary to infection in other organs. The meningococcus may also be responsible for an acute fulminating septicaemia, with adrenal haemorrhage and failure, with or without signs of meningitis. An extensive purpuric rash may precede or accompany signs of meningitis.

Acute bacterial meningitis is ushered in by headache, fever, vomiting, rapidly developing confusion, delirium, coma, twitching and convulsions. While the patient is conscious, meningismus and photophobia may be prominent.

Diagnosis

Lumbar puncture should be carried out without delay in all patients with clinical signs of meningitis. The CSF in bacterial meningitis is nearly always under increased pressure and cloudy in appearance. Microscopy shows a raised polymorphonuclear leukocyte count, and there is a raised protein concentration and a low glucose concentration. The organism responsible is usually demonstrated by Gram's stain or culture.

Infection and transmission

Infection is usually from nasopharyngeal infection by droplet spread.

Incubation period

For meningococcal meningitis this is 3–5 days.

Prevention

Outbreaks of meningococcal infection occur most often in over-crowded conditions such as army barracks. Contacts should be treated immediately with prophylactic sulphonamide, rifampicin or minocycline. Acute meningitis is a notifiable disease.

Treatment

Meningococcal meningitis may present as a fulminating condition and treatment may be necessary before the organism has been identified or the patient transferred to hospital. In such cases 600 mg of crystalline penicillin intravenously or intramuscularly every 4 hours with 100 mg of hydrocortisone may be life-saving. In addition, some patients may benefit from crystalline penicillin intrathecally. Subsequent antibiotic therapy in all cases depends upon the identification and sensitivities of the organism.

Diphtheria

Diphtheria is an acute infection of the nasopharynx caused by *Corynebacterium diphtheriae*. The characteristic lesion is the adherent membrane which is not confined to the tonsils. The exotoxin can have a profound systemic effect on the myocardium or the central nervous system. Once a scourge of childhood, diphtheria is now rare as a result of immunization (see Chapter 3, p. 39). If suspected, urgent hospital admission must be arranged for treatment with antitoxin.

Tetanus

Tetanus is a notifiable disease carrying a high mortality. It is caused by a spore-forming anaerobic bacillus, *Clostridium tetani,* which lives in soil and animal faeces, particularly horses'. The bacillus or its spores enter the skin through a puncture wound, and the multiplication of the bacilli and production of the powerful exotoxin are encouraged by the presence of devitalized tissue. The first symptom is usually spasms of muscles in the locality of the wound, followed by paroxysms of muscle spasm superimposed on a generalized tonic rigidity. This most often affects the masseters, hence the synonym lockjaw.

The incubation period varies from 2 days to about 3 weeks, and in general the longer the incubation period the better the prognosis. Tetanus can be prevented by active immunization (see Chapter 3, p. 39). At the time of an injury the use of toxoid or immunoglobulin, where indicated, must be accompanied by thorough cleaning and debridement of wounds. The treatment of established cases requires hospital care as tracheostomy and artificial ventilation may be necessary in addition to antibiotics and antitoxin.

Whooping cough (pertussis)

Whooping cough is a respiratory infection caused by *Bordetella pertussis* and characterized by a paroxysmal cough and whoop.

Symptoms

A catarrhal stage lasting about a week is followed by a period of increasing spasmodic cough. Fever is mild or absent. During a spasm a series of uncontrollable coughing efforts occur with no respite to snatch a breath. The face becomes suffused; saliva, mucus and vomitus are exuded. The spasm over, the first massive breath sucked in causes the characteristic whoop. The patient is usually remarkably well between spasms. Over the next 2 weeks the spasms gradually become less frequent and less severe, and the illness usually lasts about a month in all. Whooping is uncommon in adolescents and adults. Mild attacks of whooping cough are frequently seen in those who have been immunized against the disease. Complications are uncommon in children of school age but may be dangerous in infancy.

Diagnosis

The clinical suspicion may be confirmed by bacteriological examination of a pernasal swab.

Incubation period

7 – 10 days.

Period of communicability

Whooping cough may be transmitted for as long as a month after onset of the catarrhal stage, and those most at risk of serious illness are the youngest siblings of the patient.

Immunity

An attack confers prolonged immunity.

Prevention

Immunization (see Chapter 3, p. 40) is the most effective means of prevention. Whooping cough is a notifiable disease which continues to be a dangerous infection to infants, so special efforts must be made to protect them. Parents should always be notified of cases occurring in a school and advised to take appropriate precautions with this in mind. The period of communicability can be reduced by giving erythromycin, so its main indication is to reduce the risk of transmission to infant contacts.

Treatment

Whooping cough is an unpleasant, prolonged illness where good nursing is of most help to the patient. The place of antibiotics is controversial. If they are used, erythromycin or co-trimoxazole are most likely to be of use.

Return to school

A pupil should not return until at least 3 weeks after the onset of paroxysmal cough, and then only if clinically recovered.

Tuberculosis

Tuberculosis is now uncommon in the UK, where it is usually an imported disease. Primary tuberculosis of the lungs is usually self-limiting and symptomless but detectable by X-ray examination and subsequent conversion of the skin reaction to tuberculin. In complicated cases pleural effusions, segmental collapse of a lobe, gland rupture, tuberculous bronchopneumonia and miliary tuberculosis may occur. This occasionally leads to tuberculous meningitis, in which the symptoms develop slowly but proceed inexorably until treatment is instituted. Tuberculosis of bone and lymphatic tissue is now rare.

Postprimary or adult infection of the lungs leads to variable chronic inflammation and destruction of lung tissue, and these patients are the usual source of infection.

Tuberculosis is a notifiable disease. When an open case of tuberculosis occurs, contact-tracing and isolation of the patient are important public health measures. Because of the risk of transmission of tubercle bacilli from adult postprimary cases to children, staff working in schools should be screened radiologically (see Chapter 2, p. 19). BCG vaccination of schoolchildren is recommended as national policy in the prevention of tuberculosis (see Chapter 3, pp. 42-3).

Conjunctivitis

Infective conjunctivitis may be caused by a wide variety of bacterial and viral agents, and may be difficult to distinguish from allergic conjunctivitis which is especially common in the hay fever season.

Mucopurulent conjunctivitis is of importance in schools as it can spread rapidly through direct contact and communal towels. There is catarrhal inflammation of one or both eyes, with conjunctival infection, and a variable amount of discharge; the discharge is thin and slight at first, later becoming mucopurulent and occasionally purulent. Exclusion from school is only necessary for younger children and in very acute cases. Personal hygiene and the use of personal towels all help to reduce transmission. Culture is seldom very informative, and the best treatment is chloramphenicol eye drops during the day, and the same drug in ointment form at night (because of its prolonged effect and assistance in preventing the eyelids sticking together).

Brucellosis

Brucellosis is an infectious disease caused by *Brucella abortus, suis* or *melitensis,* exhibiting a febrile stage without specific clinical features and a chronic stage characterized by relapses of fever, malaise, sweating, lassitude and headache. It is now rare in the UK following its virtual elimination from dairy herds and the wide-spread practice of pasteurizing milk.

Weil's disease (leptospiral jaundice)

This comparatively rare cause of hepatitis is usually seen among sewage workers, fishermen and farm labourers. It is due to the *Leptospira icterohaemorrhagica* or more rarely *L. canicola*. The infection is usually transmitted through the urine of infected rats or dogs contaminating food and bathing places. Hospital admission is necessary for investigation and treatment with antibiotics.

Intestinal infections

Food poisoning

Food poisoning is a disease which must be notified on suspicion whatever the cause. An acute inflammation of the lining of the stomach and intestine results from the ingestion of infected or contaminated food. The causal agent may be:

(a)   bacterial, e.g. *Salmonella, Clostridium welchii, B. cereus*.

(b)   bacterial toxins, e.g. staphylococcal enterotoxin, botulinum toxin.

(c)   non-bacterial, e.g. fungal, chemical (including pesticides, which usually cause neurological symptoms).

Diagnosis is by isolation of the causal agent from the food, faeces or vomitus.

Mass outbreaks in schools or parties are suggestive of food poisoning due to bacteria or bacterial toxins. In such cases the outbreak may be explosive, occurring within a few hours of ingestion of the contaminated food. Food may be contaminated by handlers with infected wounds, nasopharyngeal discharges or enteric infections. Bacterial contamination may occur in raw, inadequately cooked, and reheated food. The staphylococcus produces a heat-stable enterotoxin which may resist cooking. (See also Chapter 2, pp. 18–19).

In *B. cereus* food poisoning the source is rice which has either been boiled in bulk and stored under warm conditions before reheating, or fried for a short time with freshly beaten egg. Nausea and vomiting are the predominant symptoms.

Incubation periods

These vary according to the degree of contamination. Staphylococcal food poisoning due to enterotoxin has a more rapid onset than types due to bacterial infection. The following periods are a rough guide:

Staphylococcus	½–6 hours (usually 1–2 hours)
B. cereus	½–11 hours (usually 1½–4 hours)
Salmonella	6–48 hours (usually 12–24 hours)
Cl. welchii	8–24 hours (usually 10–12 hours)

Prevention

Food poisoning is best prevented by attention to the principles of hygiene described in Chapter 2. Outbreaks should be fully investigated by the local environmental health department or the Public Health Laboratory Service (see Appendix A, pp. 182–6).

Treatment

The most important, and often the only, component of treatment for most forms of gastroenteritis is fluid replacement. A suitable solution can be made up of a pinch of salt and a teaspoonful of sugar in 250 ml water; more sophisticated solutions are sodium chloride and glucose oral powder, compound, and similar preparations listed in the British National Formulary. Kaolin or codeine phosphate may relieve the diarrhoea, and antiemetics such as metoclopramide may be given if vomiting is severe. Antibiotics are of no help and are specifically contraindicated as they may prolong the carrier state and aggravate diarrhoea by altering the intestinal flora.

Return to school

Pupils may return to school on clinical recovery. In cases of salmonellosis a negative stool should ideally be obtained before return to the community. This rule may have to be relaxed for prolonged excretors, who must nevertheless be excluded from all food handling until three successive negative stools have been obtained.

Bacillary dysentery

Bacillary dysentery is a notifiable disease caused by the Shigella group of organisms. In Britain *S. sonnei* accounts for over 90% of cases, and *S. flexneri* for most of the rest. Classically, it is characterized by diarrhoea of acute onset, with fever, blood and mucus in the stools, colic and tenesmus. The majority of infections, however, are mild and many are symptomless. Young children are particularly susceptible, and outbreaks can be particularly troublesome in nursery schools and residential children's homes. The diagnosis is made by stool culture or rectal swab.

The source of infection is from excreta of patients or carriers, the route being faecal–oral directly or through contaminated food, toilets, eating utensils and, rarely, water. Flies may act as vectors.

Incubation period

This is usually 2–4 days, but may be 1–7 days.

Period of communicability

Dysentery may be transmitted as long as the organisms persist in the faeces. This is usually days or weeks, but a carrier state may persist for months.

Prevention

Prevention is by attention to hygiene. Contacts should be instructed in strict hand hygiene.

Treatment

Severe cases in infants require hospitalization for correction of dehydration and electrolyte disturbance. Ordinary acute cases require bed rest, fluids and symptomatic treatment. Antibiotics such as co-trimoxazole should be reserved for severe cases.

Return to school

Pupils may return to school after two successive negative stool cultures, but the return of the persistent carrier calls for special consideration. Symptomless carriers are not highly infectious and play little part in the spread of an outbreak, unless engaged in handling food.

Management of an outbreak

'It is a golden rule in the investigation of any outbreak of infection never to take any swabs until one has decided what to do with the positives'. Christie[4] discusses the problems of managing an outbreak in an institution and the reader faced with this situation is referred to his book.

Amoebic dysentery

This is not an indigenous infection in the UK. It is caused by the *Entamoeba histolytica* and usually presents as a colitis with bloody mucoid stools, but late forms such as amoebic hepatitis may occur. Diagnosis and treatment are difficult, and should be carried out where possible by a tropical diseases hospital.

Gastroenteritis

A large number of organisms cause diarrhoea and vomiting, which may occur in epidemic form in schools. Dysentery and food poisoning, including Salmonella infection, have been dealt with above. Other causes of intestinal infection are as follows:

Campylobacter jejuni

Campylobacter organisms, only known as human pathogens since 1977, cause more cases of diarrhoea in the UK than salmonellae. The source is most commonly inadequately cooked poultry and unpasteurized milk, as the organism is readily destroyed by heat. Cases occur sporadically and also in large outbreaks. Schools outbreaks have been traced to unpasteurized milk and in one case to a contaminated water supply. The incubation period is usually from 3–5 days, and abdominal pain and fever often precede diarrhoea. The pain may be sufficiently severe and prolonged to mimic appendicitis. Vomiting is uncommon, but the diarrhoea may persist for several days. Diagnosis is by isolation of the organism from the stools. Spread from human to human rarely occurs except in young children. Although erythromycin is effective *in vitro*, it is seldom necessary, as the disease is self-limiting.

Yersinia enterocolitica

Y. enterocolitica is another organism which has only come to attention in recent years[5] and has been implicated in school outbreaks. It causes mesenteric adenitis with abdominal pain and fever. Diarrhoea is commoner in young children than in adolescents. Transmission is by the faecal–oral route, and an important feature may be that the organism can proliferate in contaminated food at temperatures as low as 4°C.

E. coli

Enterotoxic strains of *E. coli* cause infantile gastroenteritis, and traveller's diarrhoea.

Viruses

A number of viruses are responsible for gastrointestinal infections, and may be identified by electron microscopy. Enteroviruses cause minor gastrointestinal symptoms. Rotaviruses cause extensive outbreaks, most commonly in young children. Winter vomiting disease occurs in explosive outbreaks in boarding schools, and appears to be caused by parvoviruses, of which the Norwalk agent is one.

Giardia lamblia

Giardia lamblia is a protozoon which causes persistent traveller's diarrhoea. It is endemic, for example, in Leningrad. The diagnosis is made by microscopy of the stools, and metronidazole is effective treatment: 2 g per day for 3 days or 400 mg t.d.s. for 7 days.

Typhoid and paratyphoid fever

Typhoid and paratyphoid are caused by *Salmonella typhi A, B and C*.

Typhoid is widespread throughout both temperate and tropical zones, particularly in areas with poor sanitation and hygiene. While local residents in endemic areas may exhibit a high degree of immunity, the unprotected traveller is at special risk. Most cases in Britain in recent years have been in persons infected on holiday abroad; indigenous infection is rare in the UK.

Typhoid is a systemic illness of insidious onset characterized by a slowly rising fever, bradycardia, rose spots on the abdomen and back, splenomegaly and an apathetic mental state. Constipation is common in the early stages and may be followed by diarrhoea. In the later stages in the untreated case, bowel haemorrhage, perforation and peritonitis may occur and need prompt treatment. Blood culture is the most important early diagnostic method. Culture of urine and faeces and the Widal agglutination test may also be helpful.

The source of the organism is the faeces or urine of a patient or carrier. Food and milk contaminated by an infected handler, water from a contaminated source, fly-borne infection, or inadequately sterilized canned food may be responsible for outbreaks of typhoid.

The epidemiology of paratyphoid is similar to that of typhoid fever except that it is nearly always food-borne.

Incubation period

Usually 10–14 days.

Period of communicability

Patients, after clinical recovery, may excrete *S. typhi* in the urine and faeces for many years. Therefore, any patient is a potential source of infection for as long as the organism can be cultured from the urine or faeces.

Prevention

Typhoid and paratyphoid are notifiable diseases. Prevention is by good hygiene and avoidance of raw food and water in endemic areas. Travellers to these areas should have typhoid vaccine (see Chapter 3, p. 46).

Treatment

Chloramphenicol is the most effective antibiotic, but in view of the risks of its toxic effects some practitioners prefer to use co-trimoxazole.

Return to school

Patients may return to school when clinically fit and after at least three successive negative faecal and urine cultures at 2 or 3 day intervals.

Tropical and imported diseases

Malaria

Malaria is a notifiable disease caused by a parasitic protozoon of the genus *Plasmodium*. The early development of the parasite takes place in the gut of the Anopheles mosquito, from where it passes through the salivary apparatus and is injected into the bloodstream of its human host when the female mosquito feeds. The distribution of malaria follows that of the Anopheles mosquito and is mainly confined to tropical and subtropical regions throughout the world. As the mosquito requires water for the completion of its life cycle, malaria may show a seasonal variation in incidence in regions which have a wet and a dry season.

An increasing number of cases of malaria are imported every year, and school doctors should always be alert to the possibility.

Malignant tertian malaria is caused by *P. falciparum*, benign tertian by *P. vivax* or *P. ovale*, and benign quartan by *P. malariae*. The symptoms of all types are an abrupt onset of fever with headache, joint pains, rigors, anorexia and vomiting. A pattern of remission and recurring fever develops later, but the diagnosis should be made before this is established. There are many grave complications of malignant tertian malaria.

Diagnosis

The diagnosis can be difficult. Malaria should always be suspected when a febrile illness occurs in any person who has returned from an endemic area within 1 month, or longer when antimalarial prophylaxis has been taken. Proof of infection is obtained by finding the malarial parasite in thick or thin blood films stained with Leishman's stain.

Prevention

Malarial prophylaxis is dealt with in Chapter 3, (pp. 48–9).

Treatment

The correct use of antimalarial drugs has been complicated by the development of resistant parasites. Treatment should therefore be supervised by a tropical diseases specialist.

Viral haemorrhagic fever

The viral haemorrhagic fevers, Lassa fever, Marburg disease and
Ebola fever, are diseases of West Africa and the Sudan which have
occasionally been imported into Europe with much attendant pub-
licity on account of their considerable mortality rates. They should
be thought of in cases of pyrexia of unknown origin in travellers who
have arrived from these areas within the 3 weeks preceding their
illness. If suspected, the Medical Officer for Environmental Health
should be informed immediately.

Rabies

The few occurrences of rabies in the UK are in patients who have
contracted the disease overseas. It is acquired from the bite or lick
of a rabid animal, usually a dog or cat, and is almost invariably fatal
once neurological symptoms have developed. The incubation
period is usually 2–8 weeks. A prodromal illness of headache, fever
and apprehension leads to the symptoms of cerebral irritation, with
excitement, convulsions, hypersensitivity and hydrophobia.

Rabies vaccine is dealt with in Chapter 3 (p. 47). Detailed
recommendations are given in the DHSS Memorandum on Rabies[6].
If a case is suspected, expert advice should be obtained without
delay.

Sexually transmitted diseases

All patients with sexually transmitted diseases should, if possible,
be referred to special clinics because of the need for accurate
diagnosis, the exclusion of multiple infection, appropriate treatment, follow-up and contact tracing. This applies to schoolchildren
as much as to adults, and they should be reassured about the
expertise and confidentiality with which they will be treated. Only
brief descriptions of the diseases will be given here.

Gonorrhoea

Gonorrhoea is caused by infection with the gonococcus, *Neisseria
gonorrhoeae*. The incubation period is short, usually 2–5 days, and
the presenting symptom in the male is urethritis, with dysuria and a
urethral discharge. In the female the disease is often symptomless,
but there may be dysuria and a vaginal discharge. Complications

include epididymitis in the male, and Bartholinitis and pelvic infection in the female. Contact with the gonococcus in the birth canal can cause ophthalmia neonatorum. Treatment by penicillin is very effective except when the infecting organism has developed penicillin resistance.

Non-specific urethritis

Non-specific urethritis is a common sexually-transmitted disease, probably caused by *Chlamydia trachomatis*. The incubation period is 2–3 weeks, and the symptoms of discharge and dysuria are usually less severe than in gonorrhoea. Complications include prostatitis, epididymitis and Reiter's syndrome. Treatment is more difficult than in the case of gonorrhoea, and a fairly long course of tetracycline or erythromycin is usually necessary.

Syphilis

Syphilis, a disease of historical importance and protean manifestations, is now uncommon in the UK. It is caused by infection with *Treponema pallidum,* and has an incubation period of 9–90 days. The primary lesion is the painless genital chancre. 6–8 weeks later the secondary manifestations of influenza-like symptoms and a rash appear. Diagnosis is by discovery of the treponemes in scrapings from the chancre examined microscopically with dark-ground illumination. Serological tests for syphilis become positive at a later stage. The diagnosis, treatment and follow-up must be in the hands of a special clinic.

Genital herpes

Genital herpes, caused by herpes simplex virus Type II, resembles herpes simplex of the lip. The incubation period is 4–5 days, after which a cluster of vesicles appears on the genitalia. These usually rupture and form painful erosions which heal in about 10 days unless secondarily infected. Recurrences may occur, but are usually less severe than the first attack. The disease is essentially self-limiting, but can be treated with idoxuridine solution or acyclovir cream.

Genital warts

Genital warts, or condylomata acuminata, are viral warts transmitted sexually. The incubation period is usually about 3 months. Treatment with podophyllin and similar agents is best carried out at hospital.

Trichomonas vaginalis infection

Trichomonas infection, due to a flagellated protozoon, is usually sexually acquired. In the female it is manifested by a frothy, malodorous vaginal discharge which causes irritation and soreness. In both sexes there may be dysuria. Diagnosis is confirmed by microscopy and culture. Treatment with metronidazole is nearly always effective.

Other sexually transmitted diseases

Scabies and pediculosis pubis may be transmitted sexually and are described in the section on skin infection below (p. 173). Candidiasis (vaginal thrush, due to yeast organisms) is not usually caused by sexual activity but may be transmitted sexually. Predisposing factors include diabetes, oral contraceptives, broad spectrum antibiotics and pregnancy. The symptoms are an itchy vaginal discharge and balanitis, and diagnosis is confirmed by microscopy and culture. Treatment is by the local application, in the form of pessaries or cream, of nystatin, clotrimazole, miconazole or econazole.

Skin infections

Impetigo contagiosa

Impetigo is a superficial infection of the skin initially causing vesicles, which later become crusted seropurulent plaques. The causal organism is *Streptococcus pyogenes* or *Staphylococcus pyogenes;* sometimes both together. Diagnosis is on clinical appearance and by culture of a swab from the lesion. Impetigo is acquired by contact with a case or carrier. The incubation period is short, and the lesions are highly infectious until healed.

Contacts of streptococcal impetigo may develop throat infections. Acute nephritis still commonly occurs in some tropical countries and in young children more often follows streptococcal skin infection than upper respiratory infection.

Prevention requires attention to personal hygiene as well as the prompt diagnosis and treatment of established cases. Young children and severe cases should be excluded from school in the acute stage. This is particularly necessary during an outbreak of streptococcal infection.

Treatment should be with an antibiotic cream or ointment such as chlortetracycline or fusidic acid, depending on the sensitivities of the organism. Systemic antibiotics – penicillin or erythromycin for streptococcal infections – may be needed in the more severe cases.

Erisypelas

Erisypelas is an acute infection of the skin caused by *Streptococcus pyogenes*. There is fever and an acutely inflamed erythematous swelling of the skin with a sharply defined border. The commonest site is the face. Erisypelas can occur at any age, but is commonest in the elderly. The infection responds to penicillin and erythromycin.

Scabies

Scabies is a contagious skin disease, rarely transmitted from animals, caused by the penetration of a mite, *Sarcoptes scabiei*. The characteristic burrows are to be found most commonly on the front of the wrist, the ulnar side of the hand, the webs of the fingers, the anterior axillary folds, the umbilicus and the genitalia. The face is free. Sometimes the skin over the end of the burrow is raised into a small vesicle. Itching occurs most persistently at night when the patient gets warm in bed. Cases may present simply as 'the itch' with a sparse rash.

The diagnosis is made on clinical appearance and by recognition of the mite microscopically. Transmission is generally by close and prolonged contact. The infection is usually contracted in bed from an infected companion or spread through clothing or bedding.

Scabies is treated by the application of an insecticide, which should be used by all members of the household. Benzyl benzoate application 1%, gamma benzene hexachloride cream or monosulfiram (Tetmosol) 25% in an alcoholic base, diluted with 2 or 3 parts of water, is applied from the neck down following a hot bath during which burrows are gently rubbed open with a soft brush. After treatment the patient may be allowed to return to school at once.

Pediculosis (lice)

Pediculosis is an infestation of the head, the hairy parts of the body or the clothing, by blood-sucking lice. These are *Pediculus capitis* (the head louse), *Pediculus corporis* (the body louse) and *Pediculus pubis* (the crab louse). By far the commonest of these in schools is the head louse, which has greatly increased in prevalence in recent years to the point where it is almost endemic.

The head louse exists in three forms – egg or nit, nymph, and adult. The egg is yellowish to grey-white, and is from 0.8–1.0 mm long. It is attached to a hair close to the scalp by a cement-like substance and incubated by heat. Following an incubation period of about a week the young nymph emerges and remains in the nymph stage for 8–9 days before it develops to sexual maturity. The nymph looks like an adult but does not have a fully developed reproductive capacity. The adult louse – a female – is about 3 mm long. Its body is composed of three parts: a head, thorax (with three pairs of legs), and segmented abdomen. At the end of each leg is a hook-like claw and opposing thumb, which enable the louse to maintain its hold on hair.

Symptoms

The bite of the louse causes irritation, and the principal symptom of infestation is itching. Children seen to scratch their heads repeatedly often prove to have head lice.

Diagnosis

Adults and nymphs of head lice are found on the hair and on the scalp. They are more prevalent on the back of the neck and behind the ears, because head lice prefer shaded areas to those exposed to light. Generally, a single individual will harbour only 10–20 head lice, so there are very few crawling forms on any individual. Nits are laid close to the scalp, so any found more than 1 cm from the scalp are almost certainly hatched or dead.

Period of communicability

Head lice are spread only by direct contact. Body lice can be spread by infested clothing or bedding, and crab lice are usually spread by sexual contact. Transmission can occur at any time while live lice are present.

Prevention

A national campaign to eliminate head lice by inspection and treatment of all schoolchildren in 1977 failed totally. Nevertheless, regular inspection is still carried out in schools and is worth while for the detection of cases and reduction of the risk of spread.

Treatment

Malathion and carbaryl are recommended as the best treatment for lice. The lotion should be applied to dry hair, rubbed into the scalp and removed by washing after 12 hours. It is wise to repeat the procedure after 7–9 days. Gamma benzene hexachloride has fallen out of favour because of the supposed emergence of resistant strains.

In the case of body lice, heating to 55°C for 40 minutes will kill lice and eggs in clothing and other fomites.

Return to school

Pupils can return to school after effective treatment.

Ringworm

This is a general term applied to certain mycotic infections of the keratinized areas of the body, i.e. hair, skin and nails. The lesions are caused by dermatophytes, some of which are found in domestic and wild animals who act as sources of infection for man. Dogs are often the source of infection for children. *Microsporon canis* is the common cause of ringworm in cats and dogs and is easily transmitted to man. Cattle ringworm causes unusually inflammatory lesions in man: the characteristic scalp condition is known as kerion. Where there is clinical uncertainty, confirmation of the diagnosis of ringworm should be sought by microscopy and culture of scrapings or nail clippings.

Tinea pedis ('Athlete's foot')

There are two types of this common infection, the acute inflammatory condition and the more usual chronic dry type. The acute type arises in the toe-clefts, usually between the 4th and 5th toes, and may spread over the feet causing a vesiculo-pustular eruption. The principal symptom of the dry type is itching.

Tinea cruris ('Dhobie itch')

Tinea of the groin occurs predominately in males, and must be distinguished from simple intertrigo. It is usually bilateral and starts as a round, scaly, itchy patch on the inside of the thigh spreading peripherally from the groin, with an active advancing edge which is red and slightly scaly. Unlike intertrigo, tinea cruris usually itches.

Tinea corporis (Body ringworm)

Most species of *Trichophyton* and *Microsporon* can involve areas of smooth skin, usually producing red-ringed lesions with small peripheral vesicles and a scaly centre.

Tinea unguum (Ringworm of the nails)

Fungus infections of the toenails and fingernails produce a characteristic dystrophy of the nails which is symptomless but extremely chronic.

Tinea capitis (Scalp ringworm)

Scaly patches of different sizes with broken hairs are characteristic of scalp ringworm. The disease may spread to the eyelids, neck and trunk. The diagnosis can be made using Wood's lamp, as fluorescence occurs in most cases of scalp ringworm.

Prevention

Tinea pedis, in particular, is fairly easily spread by wet surfaces and towels. Pupils with acute tinea pedis should be excluded from swimming, and communal towels should be avoided. No other exclusion from school is needed, and control is best maintained by early treatment when infection occurs.

Treatment

A variety of topical fungicides can be used for all types of ringworm, supplemented where necessary by oral griseofulvin or ketoconazole. Whitfield's ointment (compound benzoic acid ointment) has stood the test of time and is still effective, but has now largely been superseded by more elegant proprietary preparations containing clotrimazole, econazole or miconazole. Twice daily application of one of these will clear most cases of tinea pedis, cruris and corporis. Acute weeping tinea pedis is best treated in the early stages by soaking the feet in a 1 in 8000 solution of potassium permanganate for several minutes up to 3 times a day. Scalp ringworm and some cases of nail ringworm should be treated with griseofulvin tablets in a dose of 0.5–1 g daily (or 10 mg/kg for a child). In the case of nail ringworm, especially of the toenails, the treatment needs to be prolonged and this must be weighed up in deciding whether to embark on treatment at all. Local treatment of extensive tinea corporis can be supplemented by griseofulvin for 2–3 weeks.

Candidiasis (thrush)

Thrush is caused by yeast organisms, usually *Candida albicans,* although other species may produce illness. Oral thrush is mainly a disease of infants, although some cases of stomatitis and pharyngitis in older children and adults are due to *Candida* infection. Primary infection also causes vulvo-vaginitis (see p. 89), intertrigo (including nappy rash) and chronic paronychia. Diabetics, the immunodeficient, and patients on broad spectrum antibiotic treatment are particularly at risk, and serious systemic illness sometimes occurs in patients with severe underlying diseases.

Treatment of cutaneous candidiasis, which is the only kind commonly occurring in schoolchildren, is with topical amphotericin, nystatin or one of the broad spectrum fungicides mentioned in the section on ringworm above.

Warts

Warts are caused by the human papovavirus. They may occur on any part of the body, including the genitalia (see p. 171), and are spread by direct contact. The wart virus probably enters wherever there is any minor breach of skin surface. The type which causes most concern at school is the plantar wart, or verruca plantaris. It has the same histological features as a wart on any other part of the body but to the naked eye presents a characteristically countersunk appearance. It may occur anywhere on the plantar surface of the foot but is most commonly found at sites of greatest pressure: the forepart of the sole, beneath the metatarsal heads and on the heel. The highest incidence of verrucae is at puberty, most cases occurring between 10 and 14 years.

Transmission of warts is by direct contact, presumably by virus deposited on the ground by infected persons. It is believed that plantar warts can be spread by contact with surfaces recently contaminated by the virus, as on the verges of swimming pools and the floors of changing rooms, showers and bathrooms. Several studies have shown a correlation between the use of swimming baths and plantar warts, but there is no evidence to support the popularly-held belief that barefoot physical education plays an important part in transmission. Paronychial warts are perpetuated by the repeated trauma of nail-biting, and usually persist as long as the habit itself.

Incubation period

This is long, 1–6 months.

Period of communicability

Warts are probably communicable as long as they are active.

Immunity

The immunology of warts is not yet fully worked out, but the slow development of immunity probably accounts for the spontaneous regression which eventually takes place.

Prevention

There is no justification for restrictive measures to try to prevent the spread of this almost universal self-limiting minor condition. Active lesions can be covered when swimming, but children with warts should not be excluded from swimming or barefoot activities.

Treatment

Over 95% will disappear spontaneously in time without treatment, but treatment is justified when the warts are painful. The variety of methods available testifies to their limited effectiveness. Among the keratolytic preparations, podophyllin compound paint or salicylic acid collodion, applied daily, with regular paring of the warts, are effective and almost painless. Curettage and cautery are no more likely to effect a permanent cure, and healing is slow, so they have no real place in treatment. Liquid nitrogen, however, can be helpful in intractable cases.

Worm infections

Of the many worm infections afflicting man, few occur in Europe except as exotic rarities, and this section will deal only with those which may occur in Western schoolchildren.

Threadworms

These are the commonest of worm infections in the UK. They are also known as pinworms and oxyuriasis. They may be symptomless, or cause sleep disturbance through anal and vaginal itching. The adult worm inhabits the intestine and the female lays her eggs at night in the perianal area. The male worm is 2–5 mm in size, white and threadlike in appearance, and the female is 8–13 mm long.

Diagnosis

The diagnosis is made by recognition of the worms on the buttocks or stools, or collection of ova on a perianal swab or adhesive tape.

Incubation period

3–6 weeks.

Communicability

The infection is transmitted by the faecal–oral route and reinfection is common. This may keep the infection running permanently in a family group until treatment is instituted.

Prevention

Prevention requires a high standard of hygiene including short finger-nails and measures to prevent sufferers scratching the perianal region at night.

Treatment

Piperazine in tablet form or as an elixir is effective, and should be given daily for a week. All members of the family should be treated simultaneously. Mebendazole may be used in a single dose of 100 mg.

Roundworms

Roundworm infection (ascariasis) is spread by the faecal–oral route or indirectly via ova. After ingestion, larvae escape from the eggs in the duodenum, and migrate to the lungs, where further development occurs. They then enter the bronchi, ascend the trachea, are swallowed, and thus reach the small intestine, where they reach a length of 20–25 cm.

Symptoms may be caused by an allergic reaction with eosinophilia, or by intestinal obstruction due to the worms. The diagnosis is made by identification of the live worm in faeces or vomit or of ova on microscopy.

Treatment is with piperazine or mebendazole.

Tapeworms

Tapeworms have a complicated life cycle involving other animal or fish hosts. They are segmented, and segments may be recognized in the stools. Treatment is with niclosamide.

Schistosomiasis (bilharzia)

Schistosomes have an intermediate stage in water-snails, and infection may be acquired by bathing in rivers in the tropics or Middle East. There are three different species with different geographical distribution and symptom complexes. *Schistosoma haematobium* causes bladder inflammation leading to haematuria and chronic cystitis. *Schistosoma mansoni* and *Schistosoma japonicum* both cause chronic colonic inflammation and subsequent pulmonary fibrosis. The diagnosis may be suggested by eosinophilia; it should be confirmed by serology and the identification of ova in the faeces, urine or tissue biopsy. Assessment and management of established cases is a specialized field best left to hospitals for tropical diseases.

References

1. Tyrrell, D. A. J. (1965). *Common Colds and Related Diseases*. (London: Arnold)
2. Geddes, A. M. (1983). Q Fever. *Br. Med. J.*, 287, 927
3. Payler, D. K. and Purdham, P. A. (1984). Influenza A prophylaxis with amantidine in a boarding school. *Lancet*, 1, 502
4. Christie, A. B. (1980). *Infectious Diseases: Epidemiology and Clinical Practice*. 3rd Edn., pp. 118–119. (Edinburgh: Churchill Livingstone)
5. Anonymous (1984). Yersiniosis today. *Lancet*, 1, 84
6. Department of Health and Social Security (1977). *Memorandum on Rabies*. (London: HMSO)

APPENDIX A

Incubation and exclusion periods for the commoner communicable diseases

Disease	Incubation period (days)	Return to school (subject to clinical recovery)
Chickenpox	11–21 (commonly 16)	6 days after appearance of rash
Measles	10–15 (commonly 10 to onset of illness and 14 to appearance of rash)	7 days after appearance of rash
Mumps	14–18 (commonly 18)	After all swellings have subsided, usually 7–10 days
Rubella	14–21 (commonly 18)	4 days after appearance of rash
Whooping cough (Pertussis)	7–10	21 days from onset of paroxysmal cough

No routine quarantine of contacts is advised for these diseases

Table of notifiable diseases

The following diseases are notifiable to the proper officer of the local authority, who is usually the Medical Officer for Environmental Health or the District Community Physician.

Acute encephalitis	Ophthalmia neonatorum
Acute meningitis	Paratyphoid fever
Acute poliomyelitis	Plague
Anthrax	Rabies
Cholera	Relapsing fever
Diphtheria	Scarlet fever
Dysentery (amoebic or bacillary)	Smallpox
Infective jaundice	Tetanus
Lassa fever	Tuberculosis
Leprosy	Typhoid fever
Leptospirosis	Typhus
Malaria	Viral haemorrhagic fever
Marburg disease	Whooping cough
Measles	Yellow fever

To this list should be added any disease made notifiable in the area by an order made under Section 147 of the Public Health Act 1936 as amended by and construed in accordance with Section 52 of the Health Services and Public Health Act 1968 and as amended by Schedule 14 and Schedule 29, paragraph 4, to the Local Government Act 1972.

The Public Health Laboratory Service

The Public Health Laboratory Service (PHLS) is established under various National Health Service Acts for the diagnosis and the control or prevention of communicable diseases in England and Wales. It is managed by the PHLS Board on behalf of the Secretary of State for Social Services. The PHLS Headquarters Office is situated in Colindale, North London.

Functions of the Public Health Laboratory Service

The Public Health Laboratory Service comprises 52 regional or area laboratories distributed through England and Wales, and 23 reference and special laboratories or units, most of which are grouped in the Central Public Health Laboratory, Colindale, North

London, or at the Centre for Applied Microbiology and Research, Porton Down, Wiltshire.

The PHLS gives a routine microbiological service to several hospitals, and provides reference facilities that are available nationally. It collates information on the incidence of infection, and when necessary it institutes special enquiries into outbreaks and the epidemiology of infectious disease, although executive responsibility for their control is the statutory responsibility of local authorities. It also undertakes bacteriological surveillance of the quality of food and water for local authorities and others. The PHLS is often called upon to advise central and local government and the hospital service on many aspects of infectious disease. It maintains close contact with veterinary organizations in areas of mutual interest, and collaborates with the World Health Organization and with national laboratory and epidemiological services overseas.

Routine diagnostic microbiological service

Nearly all of the regional and area laboratories are situated in or are closely associated with hospitals, providing them with their routine clinical microbiological service. They also serve general practitioners, Medical Officers for Environmental Health and Environmental Health Officers. By means of this continuous sampling, the PHLS monitors the infections which bring patients to hospital or which attack them while they are there, as well as becoming aware of the distribution of infectious disease in the community.

Reference and special facilities

Most of the regional and some of the area PHLS laboratories carry out special tests for neighbouring PHLS and NHS laboratories. All PHLS laboratories are available to assist local hospital laboratories in investigating outbreaks of infection, if asked to do so.

Further back-up facilities are provided by the reference laboratories or units, which carry out various tests for PHLS and hospital laboratories throughout the United Kingdom. These tests usually require special expertise, techniques and facilities which it would be uneconomic or impossible to provide more widely. As well as carrying out special tests such as the 'fingerprinting' of organisms for epidemiological purposes, reference laboratories conduct research and act as sources of advice on many aspects of the control of communicable disease. They are consulted by other laboratories, hospital clinicians and administrators.

The PHLS special laboratories develop and produce therapeutic, prophylactic and diagnostic materials for use by the NHS and others, as well as by the Service itself. They also monitor commercially available reagents and provide test material to PHLS and hospital laboratories to enable them to assess the quality of their routine performance. The National Collection of Type Cultures is a constituent part of the Central Laboratory at Colindale.

Disease surveillance and control

A special unit, the Communicable Disease Surveillance Centre (CDSC), analyses information about the whole range of infectious diseases from the regular reports they receive from PHLS and hospital laboratories. These data form a continuously changing, up-to-date picture of communicable disease throughout the country. This is published weekly in the *Communicable Disease Report,* which is issued to microbiologists, community physicians and others concerned with disease control, supplementing information available from statutory notifications and other sources. In addition to gathering information, the Centre co-ordinates the investigation and control of incidents of communicable disease of national importance and of outbreaks involving more than one local authority. CDSC collaborates with MOSA in the collection and analysis of data on the incidence of illness in boarding schools. There is a simple weekly reporting system and analyses of the returns are sent out to participating members. More detailed reports are prepared every term. New participants are welcome, and it is suggested that all boarding school medical officers should consider taking part.

A unique feature of the PHLS is its ability, at short notice, to call on the very wide range of knowledge and ability available among its nationally distributed specialist staff. Working parties with appropriate skills can thus be formed to tackle new problems as they arise, achieving the highest probability of producing a speedy and useful result. There have been several examples of this system operating in recent years, to the considerable benefit of the community.

The Epidemiological Research Laboratory undertakes surveillance of the effectiveness and safety of many of the immunization programmes in current use, and evaluates new immunization procedures.

Research

Most PHLS laboratories are engaged in some research, and many regional laboratories, as well as the reference and special laboratories, have extensive research programmes. The Service has a number of committees which organize collaborative research projects and arrange for the testing of new ideas or methods.

Surveillance of food and drink

All regional and area laboratories provide a microbiological service to local authorities for the examination of water, milk and, increasingly, other foodstuffs, including imported foods examined at the port of entry or centre of distribution. Raw foods, in particular meat and poultry, and animal feeds known to spread agents of food poisoning, are monitored to trace the origin and transmission of these organisms. Food-poisoning bacteria are studied in relation to their survival or multiplication in foods and preventive measures are suggested in the light of results. Laboratories are often called on to examine foodstuffs in the course of investigating outbreaks of infection and they may be invited to advise manufacturers.

Arrangements for receipt of specimens

The material examined in PHLS laboratories comprises 'clinical' specimens (throat swabs, blood, faeces, etc.) from persons suspected of suffering from a microbial disease, or of being carriers of pathogenic microbes, and non-clinical ('sanitary') specimens, such as food and water, submitted either as part of an epidemiological investigation or for routine public health surveillance. No charge is made.

Clinical specimens must be submitted by medical practitioners, veterinarians, dentists, or those acting directly on their behalf.

Inquiries about services offered by PHLS laboratories should be addressed to the director of the nearest laboratory of the Service. A list of laboratories is given below.

Regional and area PHLS laboratories

Bath
Birmingham
Brighton
Bristol
Cambridge
Cardiff
Carlisle

Carmarthen
Chelmsford
Chester
Coventry
Dorchester
Epsom
Exeter
Gloucester
Guildford
Hereford
Hull

Ipswich
Leeds
Leicester
Lincoln
Liverpool
London
   Central Middlesex
       Hospital
   Dulwich
   Tooting
   Whipps Cross
Luton
Manchester
Maidstone
Middlesbrough
Newcastle
Norwich
Nottingham
Oxford

Peterborough
Plymouth
Poole
Portsmouth
Preston
Reading
Rhyl

Salisbury
Sheffield
Shrewsbury
Southampton
Stoke-on-Trent
Swansea
Taunton
Truro
Watford
Wolverhampton

The addresses of these laboratories can be found in local telephone directories.

Central Public Health Laboratory, Colindale Avenue,
London NW9 (Tel. 01-205 7041).

Communicable Disease Surveillance Centre,
61 Colindale Avenue, London NW9 5EQ (Tel. 01-200 6868).

APPENDIX B

Medical questionnaire on entry of pupil

The following questionnaire is designed to cover the salient points of importance in the pupil's medical history. Medical officers may wish to adapt it to their individual needs, adding where necessary further questions on family and social history, and such other information as may be needed for administrative purposes.

Name of pupil (BLOCK LETTERS, surname first and underline christian name by which known at home)

....

Date and place of birth ....

Has he/she had the following infections? If so, please give approximate dates:

Mumps.. Whooping cough ....

Chickenpox.................................... Rheumatic fever ....

Measles ....

Please give details of immunization against the following diseases:

	Primary course Tick appropriate box		Booster dates
	Yes	No	
Diphtheria			
Tetanus			
Pertussis (whooping cough)			
Poliomyelitis			

	Yes	No	Dates of all immunizations given
Measles			
Rubella (German measles)			
Mumps			
Typhoid			
Cholera			
Yellow fever			
Tuberculosis (BCG)			
Influenza			
Any other disease			

Has he/she required treatment for any of the following conditions?

	Yes	No
Asthma		
Eczema		
Hay fever		
Bone or joint disease		
Fits or convulsions		
Discharging ears		
Deafness		
Frequent sore throats		
Nasal obstruction		
Psychological problems		

Please give details of illness and treatment:

....

....

Please give details of any other illness, operation or hospital investigation:

....

....

Please give details of any known allergy, including sensitivity to drugs:

....

....

Has he/she lived overseas? If so, please state country and give details of any infection with tropical disease:

....

....

Please give details of any known exposure to active pulmonary tuberculosis:

....

....

Does he/she wear spectacles? ....

When was the eyesight last tested? ....

Has the colour vision been tested? ....

  If so, with what result? ....

Has he/she had an audiometry test? ....
  If so, please give date and result (pass or fail)

....

Does he/she wet the bed or have poor bladder or bowel control? ....

Please give details ....

....

Is there any feature in the family history which might have a bearing on his/her health, including any family history of psychiatric illness, coronary heart disease, high blood pressure or diabetes in the immediate family?

....

....

....

Is there any feature of his/her physical or mental health which you feel the school doctor should be aware of, or which you would like to discuss with him?

....

....

....

Do you consider that he/she is fit to take part in all the normal school games and activities?

....

Is he/she at present under any form of medical treatment?
(If yes, a letter from the specialist or family doctor would be useful.)

....

....

Signature of parent or guardian ....

Address ....

....

Telephone number: Home ....

                             Office ....

Date ....

Advice to parents of boarding school pupils

The following is suggested as a specimen notice to parents of children in boarding school.

Holiday treatment

If your son or daughter should need treatment during the holidays, they may go with their medical card to the family doctor, who will accept them as temporary patients.

If your son or daughter has an operation, accident, severe illness, immunization or special treatment during the holidays, it is necessary to inform the school medical officer on or before their return to school. The information should be given in a letter from the parent, supported if necessary by a report from the family doctor, and including details of medicines and treatment recommended, if these are to continue.

Infectious diseases

If your son or daughter is exposed during the holidays to anyone suffering from an infectious disease (e.g. chickenpox or mumps) they may return to school when the term begins, but the medical officer should be informed if your child has not already had the disease. Only in the unlikely event of contact with diphtheria, poliomyelitis, typhoid or paratyphoid fever, bacillary dysentery or meningococcal infection should the pupil be kept at home until you have consulted the school medical officer.

Tropical diseases

It is important that the school medical officer should be informed if a pupil has been exposed to the risk of malaria or other tropical disease.

Consent form

The following is suggested as a specimen consent form allowing the
medical officer to carry out immunizations and the head teacher to
act *in loco parentis* in an emergency (see also p. 35). For conveni-
ence, instruction on private treatment and participation in an accident scheme are included in the same form. The exact wording is of
course a matter for individual schools to decide.

I agree that the school medical officer may carry out such
immunizations against tetanus, poliomyelitis, measles and
rubella (German measles) as he deems necessary.

I understand that in an emergency every effort will be made to
obtain my consent to an operation and/or administration of an
anaesthetic, but if this proves impossible I hereby authorize
the headmaster or headmistress or their senior deputy to act
in loco parentis.

I wish to participate in the school's accident insurance
scheme, and will pay such premiums as are currently in force.

In the event of referral of my child to a consultant, I should like
this to be done under the National Health Service/as a private
patient. (Delete as appropriate)

Date .... *Signed* ....
                                            Parent or Guardian

APPENDIX C

The Education (School Premises) Regulations 1981

The main provision of the regulations[1] are as follows. Supplementary advice not detailed in the regulations is printed in parentheses.

Teaching accommodation

The minimum internal area of teaching accommodation varies according to the size of the school and the age of the pupils. The range is from 2.3 m² to 5.3 m² per pupil.

Recommended standards of acoustics, lighting, heating and ventilation are detailed in the Department of Educaton and Science's Design Note 17[2]. The main recommendations are as follows:

In daytime, daylight should be the main source of light in working areas except in special circumstances. Each teaching space should have a window area of at least 20% of the internal elevation of the external wall, and through which an adequate view out can be obtained. The lowest level of maintained illumination, whether daylight or electric light, at any point on a working plane should not be less than 150 lux and where fluorescent lighting is used the general level of illumination should not be less than 300 lux.

The heating system should be capable of heating a minimum of 10 m³ of fresh air per person per hour and the following resultant temperatures at a height of 0.5 m above floor level should be maintained during normal hours of occupation when the external temperature is −1°C:

21°C in areas where occupants are lightly clad and inactive (e.g. medical inspection rooms),

18°C in areas where there is an average level of clothing and inactivity (e.g. classrooms),
15°C in dormitories,
14°C in areas where the occupants are lightly clad and where activity is vigorous (e.g. gymnasia).

The temperature in circulation spaces should not be more than 3°C below the temperature of the spaces they serve.

All working areas, halls, sick rooms and dormitories should be capable of being ventilated at a minimum rate of 30 m³ of fresh air per hour for each person normally occupying these areas, or such higher rates as may be necessary to maintain comfortable conditions. Adequate measures should be taken to prevent condensation in, and to remove noxious fumes from, every kitchen and other room in which there may be steam or fumes. All lavatory accommodation, changing areas and cloakrooms in which adequate cross-ventilation to give at least six air changes per hour cannot be achieved by natural means should be mechanically ventilated.

Sleeping accommodation

Separate dormitories should be provided for boys and girls over the age of 8 years. The size of each dormitory should be kept as small as practicable.

The floor area of any dormitory should be not less than 5 m² for the first two beds, with not less than 4.2 m² for each additional bed. There should be not less than 900 mm between two beds. Cubicles should each have a window and a floor area of at least 5 m². Single bedrooms should have a minimum area of 6 m². (Bunk beds may be provided to meet a temporary need but have many disadvantages. Care must be taken to ensure adequate ventilation and to see that the bunks are structurally secure.)

Washing and sanitary provisions

In a boarding school there should be:

for every ten pupils, one bath;
for the first 60 pupils, one washbasin to every three pupils;
for the next 40 pupils, one washbasin to every four pupils;
for every additional five pupils, one washbasin;
for every five pupils, one water-closet.

Three-quarters of the number of baths may be replaced by showers.

WCs should be readily accessible from dormitories, and wash-basins should be available near to them. (A regular supply of clean towels, disposable paper towels, or electric hand-driers should be available near hand basins. Roller towels are potentially dangerous and have caused tragedies in schools: they are therefore not recommended. In accommodation for older girls, there should be privacy in washing facilities. Bins and paper bags should be pro-vided for the disposal of used sanitary towels in each WC compart-ment and suitable arrangements made for final disposal. Small electric, or preferably gas, incinerators may also be provided.)

In a day school there should be a washbasin and a WC for every ten pupils under 5 and for every 20 pupils over 5 (but with a minimum of four of each); in boys' accommodation up to two-thirds the number of WCs may be replaced by urinals.

Recreation rooms, common rooms and studies

The regulations require that living accommodation (including study bedrooms and cubicles) should be provided on a scale of not less than 2.3 m² floor area per pupil. (Separate common rooms for different age groups and sexes should be provided and a library or a quiet room should be available for more peaceful relaxation. Hobby rooms and workshops, with proper facilities and safeguards, should also be available to the pupils.)

Other provisions

The regulations state that schools must also provide facilities for storing and drying pupils' clothing. A boarding school must include an airing room, a sewing room and storage accommodation for bedding, and pupils' personal belongings. There must be separate dining and living accommodation for staff, and all schools must provide separate staff cloakrooms and washrooms.

References

1. Statutory Instrument No. 909 (1981). *The Education (School Premises) Regulations 1981*. (London: HMSO)
2. Department of Education and Science (1981). Design Note 17. *Guidelines for Environmental Design and Fuel Conservation in Educational Buildings*. (London: DES)

APPENDIX D

Swimming pool disinfectants

Chlorine-based disinfectants

Two alternatives to chlorine gas are recommended, and are in common use. The choice is between one of the chlorinated isocyanurates (such as Fi-chlor granules or tablets) and sodium hypochlorite (so-called liquid chlorine).

When the chlorinated isocyanurates are in solution, an equilibrium reaction is established between the donor molecule, cyanuric acid, and hypochlorous acid. This has the effect of prolonging the action of the disinfectant. This equilibrium reaction is particularly useful in open air pools as it has the effect of protecting free chlorine residuals against sunlight which quickly destroys them. The isocyanurates are convenient to use and store but are more expensive than sodium hypochlorite. The large demand for chlorine by high bathing loads may result in unacceptably high levels of cyanuric acid, which therefore need to be monitored. This is easily done by a bathside check with the necessary test gear.

Sodium hypochlorite is inexpensive, but if it is to be used as the only disinfectant a storage tank is needed, and the hypochlorite deteriorates if stored for long.

A convenient system is to use an isocyanurate for normal pool conditions, and to boost the free chlorine residual by means of a dosing pump and carboys of sodium hypochlorite when high bathing loads occur.

Some schools successfully use calcium hypochlorite, which like sodium hypochlorite is inexpensive. A minor disadvantage is that it is not fully soluble, and therefore has to be dosed via a settling tank and then a reservoir. It also has the disadvantage that pool staff sometimes dislike handling the powder.

Non-chlorine-based disinfectants

In general, bromine-based disinfectants are more expensive and have a weaker disinfectant action than equivalent chlorine-based compounds. They also have long-term and short-term side-effects. There is no easy method for estimating sodium bromide, which is one of the end products of the action of bromine disinfectants and is a cumulative CNS depressant. The equivalent chlorine end product is sodium chloride, which is harmless.

Chlorobromodimethylhydantoin (Di-halo) is associated with rashes, specially in older females. Skin problems may be very unusual in the school population, but severe when they do occur. No information is available on the toxicity of the donor molecule of Di-halo, dimethylhydantoin, and it cannot be estimated outside specialized laboratories. It is a member of the hydantoin group of chemicals which includes phenytoin. The chlorinated isocyanurates, which are used in the same way as Di-halo, do not have these disadvantages.

Pools treated with Baquacil tend to be cloudy and to foam and to have high bacterial counts. Baquacil is expensive and also non-algicidal, so that a powerful algicide is always needed in addition.

Sources of technical advice

It is difficult to obtain advice which is not commercially biased, although day to day advice and supplies of disinfectant may be obtained from a local swimming pool firm. When a new pool is planned or if an old pool has unusual problems, it is suggested that advice is obtained from one of the companies specializing in water treatment plant for large public pools. The following points may be helpful in avoiding problems.

Specialists should be involved early in the planning stages, and the plant installed should be designed for the maximum bathing load rather than the size of the pool. There is no substitute for pressure sand filters: the small high rate variety are not suitable for school pools because of their heavy bathing load. Disinfectants should always be injected before the filter as this is where infection may build up. When sodium hypochlorite is being used, the acid usually necessary for pH correction should be injected after the filter so that chlorine gas is not produced by direct mixing of acid and alkali. Dosing pumps must be fitted with cut-out devices so that they do not continue to inject chlorine into the pool when the main pump has failed. Dilution with fresh water is important. The practice of conserving warm water which has been used to backwash filters and returning it to the pool is hygienically unsound. Similarly, backwashing filters with mains water is not recommended as this also produces dilution of the pool.

Methods of working for swimming pool staff

Free and combined chlorine levels should be tested and recorded daily. This should be increased to three times a day when there are heavy bathing loads. When samples are being taken for bacteriological analysis, disinfectant and pH levels should be recorded at the same time from the same part of the pool. *E. coli* and coliforms should usually be absent from samples. The occasional presence of coliforms (not *E. coli*) is acceptable as long as the colony counts are not more than 10, and not more than 100 colonies per ml at 24 hours incubation. Filters should be operated for one hour before, one hour after and during bathing sessions. During times of high bathing loads, the plant should be operated for 24 hours a day. As pool contamination is mainly responsible for eye irritation and chlorinous odours, it may be necessary to limit bathing loads during very hot weather: also it is important to encourage the use of toilets before swimming. Pool surrounds should be kept visibly clean, and irrigated with a disinfectant solution containing approximately 200 ppm of chlorine, or according to the maker's instructions; it is not necessary to use disinfectants. Shampoos, soap and disinfectants should not be allowed to circulate back into the pool. School staff should refer to the disinfectant manufacturer's literature as well as to the Department of the Environment booklets on the safe operation of pools disinfected by different methods.

Reference

Department of the Environment (1984). *Treatment and Quality of Swimming Pool Water*. (London: HMSO)

APPENDIX E

The developmental progress of young children

The following charts, reproduced by permission of the Controller of Her Majesty's Stationery Office from Mary Sheridan's *Developmental Progress of Infants and Young Children* (1975, London: HMSO), should be read in conjunction with the introductory remarks on p. 51.

Age	Posture and large movement	Vision and fine movements
2½ years	Walks upstairs alone, but downstairs holding rail, two feet to a step. Runs well straight forward and climbs easy nursery apparatus. Pushes and pulls large toys skilfully, but has difficulty in steering them round obstacles. Jumps with two feet together. Can stand on tiptoe if shown. Kicks large ball. Sits on tricycle and steers with hands, but still usually propels with feet on ground.	Picks up pins, threads, etc., with each eye covered separately. Builds tower of seven (or 7+) cubes and lines blocks to form 'train'. Recognizes minute details in picture books. Imitates horizontal line and circle (also usually T and V). Paints strokes, dots and circular shapes on easel. Recognizes himself in photographs when once shown. Recognizes miniature toys and retrieves balls 2–⅛ inches at 10 feet each eye separately. (May also match special single letter-cards V O T H at 10 feet.)
3 years	Walks alone upstairs with alternating feet and downstairs with two feet to step. Usually jumps from bottom step. Climbs nursery apparatus with agility. Can turn round obstacles and corners while running and also while pushing and pulling large toys. Rides tricycle and can turn wide corners on it. Can walk on tiptoe. Stands momentarily on one foot when shown. Sits with feet crossed at ankles.	Picks up pins, threads, etc., with each eye covered separately. Builds tower of nine cubes, also (3½) bridge of three from model. Can close fist and wiggle thumb in imitation. Right and left. Copies circle (also V, H, T). Imitates cross. Draws man with head and usually indication of features or one other part. Matches two or three primary colours (usually red and yellow correct, but may confuse blue and green). Paints 'pictures' with large brush on easel. Cuts with scissors. (Recognizes special miniature toys at 10 feet. Performs single-letter vision test at 10 feet. Five letters.)

Hearing and speech	*Social behaviour and play*
Uses 200 or more recognizable words but speech shows numerous infantilisms. Knows full name. Talks intelligibly to himself at play concerning events happening here and now. Echolalia persists. Continually asking questions beginning 'What?', 'Where'? Uses pronouns, I, me and you. Stuttering in eagerness common. Says a few nursery rhymes. Enjoys simple familiar stories read from picture book. (6 toy test, 4 animals picture test, 1st cube test. Full doll vocabulary.)	Eats skilfully with spoon and may use fork. Pulls down pants or knickers at toilet, but seldom able to replace. Dry through night if lifted. Very active, restless and rebellious. Throws violent tantrums when thwarted or unable to express urgent needs and less easily distracted. Emotionally still very dependent upon adults. Prolonged domestic make-belief play (putting dolls to bed, washing clothes, driving motor-cars, etc.) but with frequent reference to friendly adult. Watches other children at play interestedly and occasionally joins in for a few minutes, but little notion of sharing playthings or adult's attention.
Large intelligible vocabulary but speech still shows many infantile phonetic substitutions. Gives full name and sex, and (sometimes) age. Uses plurals and pronouns. Still talks to himself in long monologues mostly concerned with the immediate present, including make-believe activities. Carries on simple conversations, and verbalizes past experiences. Asks many questions beginning 'What?', 'Where?', 'Who?'. Listens eagerly to stories and demands favourites over and over again. Knows several nursery rhymes. (7 toy test, 4 animals test, 1st or 2nd cube test, 6 "high frequency" word pictures.)	Eats with fork and spoon. Washes hands, but needs supervision in drying. Can pull pants and knickers down and up, but needs help with buttons. Dry through night. General behaviour more amenable. Affectionate and confiding. Likes to help with adult's activities in house and garden. Makes effort to keep his surroundings tidy. Vividly realized make-believe play including invented people and objects. Enjoys floor play with bricks, boxes, toy trains and cars, alone or with siblings. Joins in play with other children in and outdoors. Understands sharing playthings, sweets etc. Shows affection for younger siblings. Shows some appreciation of past and present.

Age	Posture and large movement	Vision and fine movements
4 years	Turns sharp corners running, pushing and pulling. Walks alone up and downstairs, one foot per step. Climbs ladders and trees. Can run on tiptoe. Expert rider of tricycle. Hops on one foot. Stands on one foot 3–5 secs. Arranges or picks up objects from floor by bending from waist with knees extended.	Picks up pins, thread, crumbs, etc., with each eye covered separately. Builds tower of 10 or more cubes and several 'bridges' of three on request. Builds three steps with six cubes after demonstration. Imitates spreading of hand and bringing thumb into opposition with each finger in turn. Right and left. Copies cross (also V, H, T, O). Draws man with head, legs, features, trunk, and (often) arms. Draws very simple house. Matches and names four primary colours correctly. (Single-letter vision test at 10 feet, seven letters: also near chart to bottom.)
5 years	Runs lightly on toes. Active and skilful in climbing, sliding, swinging, digging, and various 'stunts'. Skips on alternate feet. Dances to music. Can stand on one foot 8–10 secs. Can hop 2–3 yards forwards on each foot separately Grips strongly with either hand.	Picks up minute objects when each eye is covered separately. Builds three steps with six cubes from model. Copies square and triangle (also letters: V, T, H, O, X, L, A, C, U, Y). Writes a few letters spontaneously. Draws recognizable man with head, trunk, legs, arms and features. Draws simple house with door, windows, roof and chimney. Counts fingers on one hand with index finger of other. Names four primary colours and matches 10 or 12 colours. (Full nine letter vision chart at 20 feet and near test to bottom.)

Hearing and speech	*Social behaviour and play*
Speech completely intelligible. Shows only a few infantile substitutions usually k/t/th/f/s and r/l/w/y/ groups. Gives connected account of recent events and experiences. Gives name, sex, home address and (usually) age. Eternally asking questions 'Why?', 'When?', 'How?' and meanings of words. Listens to and tells long stories sometimes confusing fact and fantasy. (7 toy test, 1st picture voc. test, 2nd cube test. 6 "high frequency" word pictures.)	Eats skilfully with spoon and fork. Washes and dries hands. Brushes teeth. Can undress and dress except for back buttons, laces and ties. General behaviour markedly self-willed. Inclined to verbal impertinence when wishes crossed but can be affectionate and compliant. Strongly dramatic play and dressing-up favoured. Constructive out-of-doors building with any large material to hand. Needs other children to play with and is alternately co-operative and aggressive with them as with adults. Understands taking turns. Shows concern for younger siblings and sympathy for playmates in distress. Appreciates past, present and future.
Speech fluent and grammatical. Articulation correct except for residual confusions of s/f/th/ and r/l/w/y/ groups. Loves stories and acts them out in detail later. Gives full name, age and home address. Gives age and (usually) birthday. Defines concrete nouns by use. Asks meaning of abstract words. (12 "high frequency" picture vocabulary or word lists. 3rd cube test, 6 sentences.)	Uses knife and fork. Washes and dries face and hands, but needs help and supervision for rest. Undresses and dresses alone. General behaviour more sensible, controlled and responsibly independent. Domestic and dramatic play continued from day to day. Plans and builds constructively. Floor games very complicated. Chooses own friends. Co-operative with companions and understands need for rules and fair play. Appreciates meaning of clocktime in relation to daily programme. Tender and protective towards younger children and pets. Comforts playmates in distress.

Height and weight standard charts

The charts on pages 206–9 are derived from data compiled by
Tanner, Whitehouse and Takaishi[1], and are reproduced by permission of the publishers, Castlemead Publications, from whom supplies can be obtained. The reference numbers of the charts are as
follows:

Boys height and weight: 11A
Girls height and weight: 12A

The address of Castlemead Publications is:
Swains Mill,
4a Stane Mead,
Ware, Herts., SG12 9PY
(Telephone: 0920 66411).

Reference

1. Tanner, J. M., Whitehouse, R. H. and Takaishi, M. (1966). *Arch. Dis. Child.* 41,
    454, 615

Stages of genital development

Reproduced by permission of Blackwell Scientific Publications
from J. M. Tanner's *Growth at Adolescence* (1962).

Boys: genital development

Stage 1   Pre-adolescent. Testes, scrotum and penis are of about
          the same size and proportion as in early childhood.
Stage 2   Enlargement of the scrotum and testes. Skin of
          scrotum reddens and changes in texture. Little or no
          enlargement of penis at this stage.
Stage 3   Enlargement of penis, which occurs at first mainly in
          length. Further growth of testes and scrotum.
Stage 4   Increased size of penis with growth in breadth and
          development of glans. Testes and scrotum larger;
          scrotal skin darkened.
Stage 5   Genitalia adult in size and shape.

Girls: breast development

Stage 1   Pre-adolescent. Elevation of papilla only.
Stage 2   Breast bud stage: elevation of breast and papilla as small mound. Enlargement of areola diameter.
Stage 3   Further enlargement and elevation of breast and areola, with no separation of their contours.
Stage 4   Projection of areola and papilla to form a secondary mound above the level of the breast.
Stage 5   Mature stage: projection of papilla only, due to recession of the areola to the general contour of the breast.

Both sexes: pubic hair

Stage 1   Pre-adolescent. The vellus over the pubes is not further developed than that over the abdominal wall, i.e. no pubic hair.
Stage 2   Sparse growth of long, slightly pigmented downy hair, straight or slightly curled, chiefly at the base of the penis or along labia.
Stage 3   Considerably darker, coarser and more curled. The hair spreads sparsely over the junction of the pubes.
Stage 4   Hair now adult in type, but area covered is still considerably smaller than in the adult. No spread to the medial surface of thighs.
Stage 5   Adult in quantity and type with distribution of the horizontal (or classically 'feminine') pattern. Spread to medial surface of thighs but not up linea alba or elsewhere above the base of the inverse triangle (spread up linea alba occurs late and is rated stage 6).

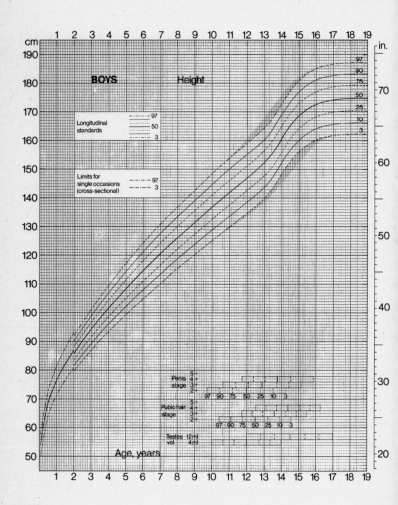

Figure 6

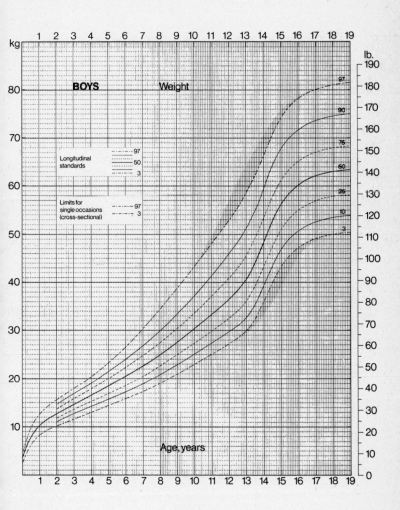

Figure 7

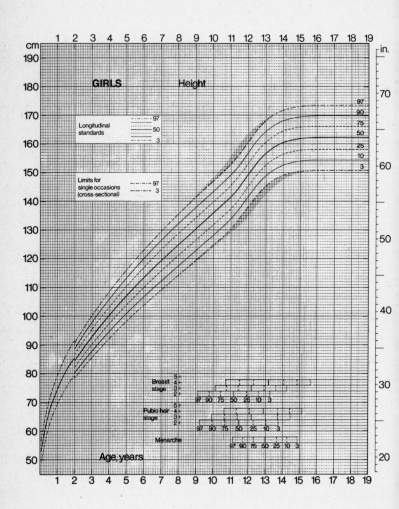

Figure 8

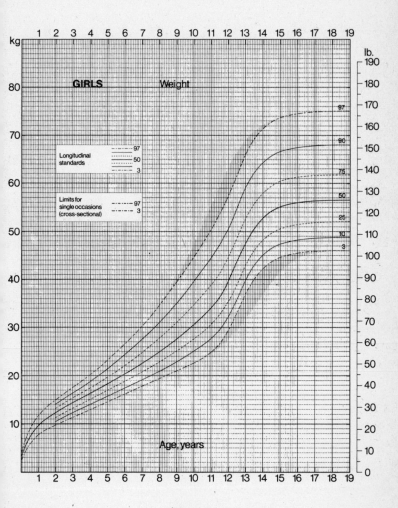

Figure 9

APPENDIX F

Colour vision

Standards of colour vision required for different occupations vary from time to time, and are published in the annual Reference Handbook of the Association of Optical Practitioners (Bridge House, 233–234 Blackfriars Road, London SE1 8NW. Telephone: 01-261 9661). The following is suggested as an information sheet for parents.

Colour Blindness

Your child ....
has been found to have defective colour vision. This condition is inherited and cannot be improved with treatment. However, it is not a great handicap except in placing some restriction on choice of career, and this should be borne in mind for the future. The careers for which defective colour vision may be a disqualification include the following:

Royal Navy Seaman officers.
Fleet Air Arm Aircrew officers.
Royal Air Force Flying personnel, photography, engineer, marine, electrical, radio, electronic, and some other branches and trades (depending on severity).
Army There are no absolute restrictions, and each case is judged on its merits. The final decision is made by the appropriate Army Medical Board.
Merchant Navy Deck officers, cadets, apprentices and ratings where look-out is required.

Railways All staff on operating duties or working among moving traffic, or involved with signal, telegraph and electrical wiring.

Civil Aviation Authority All flying personnel, air traffic controllers, most engineering apprentices.

Central Electricity Generating Board and British Telecom, etc. Those engaged in multi-coloured wiring, safety lights and warning systems.

Other careers in which defective colour vision may be a handicap include bacteriology, botany, cartography, chemistry, geology, horticulture, laboratory technician, medicine, ophthalmic optician, orthoptist, paper manufacture, paint manufacture, pharmacy, printing, textiles (dyeing and printing) and teacher of art.

If any of these careers are under consideration, further information should be obtained from the prospective employer either direct or through the Youth Employment Officer.

APPENDIX G

Sports injuries

The following tables are reprinted, with permission, from the *British Journal of Sports Medicine,* 15, 30 (Half a million hours of Rugby football, by J. P. Sparks). They show the rates of injuries recorded at Rugby School between September 1950 and December 1979.

Table 1   Injuries per 10,000 player hours

Rugby football	198
Cricket	33
Hockey	27
Cross country running	37
Athletics	26
Squash rackets	10
Rugby fives	21
Rackets	3
Lawn tennis	7
Badminton	5
Physical Education	18

Table 2   Site of injuries

Site	Injury	Number
Head	Fractured maxilla	5
	Fractured mandible	2
	Fractured nasal bones	99
	Fractured teeth	157
	Concussion	513
Chest	Fractured rib	15
	Fractured sternum	2
	Sternoclavicular subluxation	9
Abdomen	Ruptured spleen	2
	Ruptured kidney	4
	Contused scrotum	9
Spine	Fractured cervical spinous process	4
	Fractured coccyx	1
Shoulder girdle	Fractured scapula	4
	Fractured clavicle	58
	Glenohumeral dislocation	22
	Acromioclavicular subluxaton	97
Arm	Fractured neck of humerus	7
	Slipped capital humeral ephiphysis	1
	Fractured shaft of humerus	1
Elbow	Supracondylar fracture of humerus	1
	Dislocated elbow	2
	Fractured head of radius	2
Forearm	Fractured shaft of radius/ulna	8
	Colles' fracture (or greenstick)	57
	Slipped lower radial epiphysis	6
Wrist	Fractured scaphoid	7
Hand	Fractured metacarpal	39
	Fractured phalanx	183
	Dislocation – thumb – m-p jt.	6
	finger – p-i-p jt.	8
	– d-i-p jt.	8
Thigh	Fractured shaft of femur	4
	Torn quadriceps	327
	Torn hamstrings	131
	Torn adductors	73
	Calcified quadriceps haematoma	5

Knee	Tibial plateau fracture	2
	Fractured patella	1
	Dislocated patella	7
	Torn medial ligament	119
	Torn lateral ligament	14
	Torn cruciate ligament	2
	Torn medial meniscus	28
	Torn lateral meniscus	9
	Traumatic haemarthrosis	31
	Traumatic effusion	105
Shin	Fractured tibia and fibula	8
	Fractured shaft of fibula	4
Ankle	Pott's fracture	26
	Slipped lower tibial epiphysis	3
	Slipped lower fibular epiphysis	1
Foot	Fractured metatarsal	8
	Fractured phalanx	8

APPENDIX H

Specimen contract

Agreement made the ....day of
.... 19.........,
between the Governors of ABC School (or Principal where approp-
riate), (hereinafter called the School) and XYZ (hereinafter called
the Medical Officer) of

....

.... (address)

(1) For the considerations hereinafter appearing the Medical
     Officer undertakes:

    (i) To be responsible for the School Sanatorium.

    (ii) To accept as a patient under the National Health Service
     Acts any pupil attending the School as a boarder and
     receive the appropriate capitation fee.

    (iii) To visit the School not less than ...... times per week
     during school terms and whenever reasonably requested
     to do so during school holidays.

    (iv) To conduct in such manner as he shall think proper such
     routine medical examination of pupils or staff outside
     the NHS as he may consider desirable or as may be
     requested by the Governors or by the Headmaster and
     to advise the Headmaster and/or the Governors as to
     any administrative action which in his judgement should
     be taken in the interests of health or hygiene.

(v)   To make available at his own expense when requested to do so a qualified deputy, previously approved by the Governors, to act for him in cases where he is prevented from acting in person by illness or unavoidable absence.

(vi) To be and remain throughout the tenure of this Contract of Service a member of the Medical Defence Union Limited or other Medical Protection Society and to be prepared to furnish annually for the information of the Governors a certificate of membership showing the payment of the appropriate annual subscription at the due date to the organization already mentioned.

(2) In consideration of the undertakings aforesaid the School will pay the Medical Officer a capitation fee of £........ per pupil or a retaining fee of £ .... per annum to be paid termly and so long as this agreement remains in force will make available to the Medical Officer the same concessions by way of remission or partial remission of school fees in respect of any children of his who shall be attending the School as shall for the time being be accorded to members of the teaching staff.

(3) This agreement is terminable by either party giving to the other one term's (or six months') notice in writing.

(4) The salary will be reviewed annually.

(5) The date of commencement of this contract shall be
....

(6) The age of retirement of the Medical Officer shall be not less than 65, in accordance with the National Health Service.

(7) The following provisions for superannuation will apply
....

(8) In the event of any dispute arising from this contract the question shall be referred to and decided by an arbitrator to be appointed by the President of the Law Society.

Note   For those doctors who are normally employed by the school for more than 21 hours per week, the Contracts of Employment Act applies and a more detailed contract is required.

INDEX